BLUE ZONES PROJECT®
by HEALTHWAYS

Healthways CEO Ben R. Leedle Jr. has long known that the key to a healthier, happier life lies in improving more than just physical health. To truly move well-being, we have to impact individuals' sense of purpose, social connections, physical health, financial confidence, and relation to their community. When Leedle met Blue Zones® founder Dan Buettner in 2009, they quickly recognized their shared vision. In 2010, Healthways and Blue Zones joined forces to create Blue Zones Project®, a community-by-community movement to inspire people to live longer, more active lives.

Since the partnership began, Blue Zones Project has positively affected more than twenty communities across the country. In these communities, residents and business owners alike work together to improve well-being for themselves and their neighbors. The results: lower healthcare costs, improved productivity, and more socially connected people.

Today, we'd like to recognize our primary local Blue Zones Project sponsors for being our partners in innovation and community transformation. Thank you for leading the charge to create a healthier, happier world, one community at a time.

- Beach Cities, California: Beach Cities Health District
- Iowa: Wellmark Blue Cross Blue Shield
- Fort Worth, Texas: Texas Health Resources, Blue Cross Blue Shield of Texas
- Hawaii: Hawaii Medical Service Association (HMSA)
- Southwest Florida: NCH Healthcare System

We hope this book and the tales of Dan's journey are as inspiring to you as they have been for us and for Blue Zones Project communities across the country.

THE
Blue Zones
Solution

Eating and Living Like the
World's Healthiest People

Dan Buettner

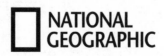

NATIONAL
GEOGRAPHIC

WASHINGTON, D.C.

Published by the National Geographic Partners
1145 17th Street NW, Washington, DC 20036

Grateful acknowledgment is made for permission to reprint "Giant Beans in Tomato Sauce" from *The Mediterranean Slow Cooker* by Michele Scicolone. Copyright © 2013 by Michele Scicolone. Reprinted by permission of Houghton Mifflin Harcourt Publishing Company. All rights reserved. Power Nine graphic (p. 20) by Blue Zones, LLC; Food Guidelines graphic (p. 164) by Joy Miller.

Library of Congress Cataloging-in-Publication Data

Buettner, Dan.
The Blue Zones solution : eating and living like the world's healthiest people / Dan Buettner.
    pages cm
Includes bibliographical references and index.
ISBN 978-1-4262-1192-8 (hardcover : alk. paper)
1. Diet. 2. Nutrition. 3. Health. 4. Functional foods. I. Title.
RA784.B75 2015
613.2--dc23

                        2014044932

National Geographic Partners
1145 17th Street NW
Washington, DC 20036-4688 USA

For information about special discounts for bulk purchases, please contact National Geographic Books Special Sales: specialsales@natgeo.com

For rights or permissions inquiries, please contact National Geographic Books Subsidiary Rights: bookrights@natgeo.com

Interior design: Melissa Farris / Katie Olsen

Printed in the United States of America

16/QGF-QGL/4

For brothers Steve, Nick, and Tony—my best friends and partners in exploration.

A MESSAGE TO THE READER

CONTENTS

FOREWORD

A S A JOURNALIST AND HEALTH ACTIVIST, Dan Buettner has redefined what it means to be a National Geographic Fellow, investigating extraordinary places around the world—called Blue Zones—where people live long, healthy lives.

In this new book, *The Blue Zones Solution,* Dan describes in detail how we can incorporate the life-extending diets and habits of these people into our own lives. Based on his extensive reporting and exhaustive research by his team of experts, Dan has teased out the key factors that have enabled Blue Zones residents to enjoy long, healthy lives. In a sense, he's reverse-engineered a solution to better health and longevity so that we, too, can live long and well.

Of course, it's not just how *long* we live, it's also how *well* we live. People in Blue Zones cultures not only live longer lives, they often live better lives, with health, meaning, and love—dying young as old as possible.

For the past several years, Dan has launched a major public health initiative to transform American cities based on principles from this book—establishing Blue Zones right here in the United States. Part of what he's learned is that you're more likely to make healthier choices when it's easier to do so. In this book, he shows you how.

His findings echo the research that my colleagues and I have conducted for almost four decades. As we've also learned, the most powerful determinants of our health and well-being are the lifestyle choices we make each day:

- Choosing a whole foods, plant-based diet (naturally low in fat and sugar)
- Practicing stress management techniques (including yoga and meditation)
- Enjoying moderate exercise (such as walking)
- Maintaining social support and community (love and intimacy, meaning and purpose)

In other words: Eat well, stress less, move more, and love more.

My colleagues and I at the nonprofit Preventive Medicine Research Institute and the University of California, San Francisco, have conducted clinical research proving the many benefits of such comprehensive lifestyle changes.

Through randomized controlled trials and other studies, we've proven the power of these simple, low-tech, and low-cost interventions and published our findings in the leading peer-reviewed medical and scientific journals.

In addition to *preventing* many chronic diseases, these comprehensive lifestyle changes can often *reverse* the progression of these illnesses.

We proved, for the first time, for example, that lifestyle changes alone can reverse the progression of even severe coronary heart disease—even more after five years than after one year, with 2.5 times fewer cardiac events. We also found that these lifestyle changes can reverse type 2 diabetes and may slow, stop, or even reverse the progression of early stage prostate cancer.

Because of this, Medicare is now covering our lifestyle program for reversing heart disease and other chronic conditions—the first time that Medicare has done so. Dan and I have partnered with Healthways to implement our visions for empowering health on a larger scale.

I often hear people say, "Oh, I've just got bad genes, there's not much I can do about it." But there is. Changing lifestyle actually changes how your genes work—turning on genes that keep you healthy, and turning off genes that promote heart disease, prostate cancer, breast cancer, and diabetes—over 500 genes in only three months.

Our latest research has also found that diet and lifestyle changes may even begin to reverse aging at a cellular level by lengthening telomeres, the ends of chromosomes that regulate aging. As your telomeres get longer, your life gets longer. And the more people adhered to these lifestyle recommendations, the longer their telomeres became.

It's not all or nothing. You have a spectrum of choices. As Dan lays out in detail in this book, what matters most is your *overall* way of eating and living.

If you indulge yourself one day, eat healthier the next. If you don't have time to exercise one day, do a little more the next. If you don't have time to meditate for 30 minutes, do it for one minute.

Just as Dan discovered in the Blue Zones, we found that the more people changed their diet and lifestyle, the more they improved and the better they felt—at any age.

—Dean Ornish, M.D.
Founder and President, Preventive Medicine Research Institute; Clinical Professor of Medicine, University of California, San Francisco; author of *The Spectrum* and *Dr. Dean Ornish's Program for Reversing Heart Disease;* www.ornish.com and www.facebook.com/ornish

INTRODUCTION

❧

Discovering the Blue Zones Solution

ONE DECEMBER AFTERNOON A FEW YEARS AGO, Bob Fagen, the 54-year-old city manager of Spencer, Iowa, pulled his SUV into the parking lot of his doctor's office. It was time for his annual physical. Lately his years of bacon-and-eggs breakfasts—and lunches that he could eat and still have one hand free to drive—had left him feeling sick and fatigued. He'd wake up tired, muscle through the day at city hall, and then, after a dinner of meat and potatoes, slump into his recliner for a few hours of yawny TV. His doctor took one look at Fagen's blood test results and said, "Bob, you need to go see a kidney specialist."

"Well, that was probably the worst thing that anybody could have said to me," Fagen said. A few years earlier, his dad had died from kidney disease, and as Fagen had watched his father hooked up to a dialysis machine, his life withering away, he'd vowed that was never going to happen to him. "Well, guess what?" Fagen said.

He kept the appointment with the specialist, his wife by his side for moral support. When the doctor looked at his blood report, he delivered the sobering news: Fagen's kidneys were failing. They were functioning at only a third of their capacity—possibly because of an allergic reaction to one of the prescription drugs Fagen was taking for diabetes, blood pressure, and cholesterol. But the specialist didn't know which one. That left them several options, he said. He could do a biopsy of Fagen's kidney to figure out what was going on. He could take Fagen off his medicines one at a time to see which was causing the trouble. Or he could take Fagen off of all of his medicines at the same time. Only one thing was certain, he explained, "If you don't get this taken care of you're not going to have a very good life from this point."

Stopping all his medicines cold turkey sounded risky to Fagen. But he was willing to give it a try if it meant getting his life back. So that's what they all agreed upon.

"As I left the office that day, I knew we were going to have to make some big changes," he said.

JUST IN TIME

Bob Fagen's story was one I'd heard before—far too many times. It was about that wake-up call you weren't expecting, telling you that life was headed in the wrong direction. People all over America, it seemed to me, were getting the same message. They were waking up to the same realization that had hit me like a slap in the face: There was something wrong about the way life was organized in this country—something about the foods we consume, the frantic pace of life we keep, the relationships we make, and the communities we create—something that keeps us from being as happy and healthy as we could be.

I knew this because, for more than a decade, I'd been traveling the world, meeting people who actually enjoyed happy, healthy lives all the way to 100—people who lived in areas we call the Blue Zones. I'd been working with a team of brilliant researchers to figure out what could explain their longevity: good genes, special diet, optimal habits? Over time, through rigorous scientific research, including fieldwork, we identified a core list of lifestyle practices and environmental factors shared among the people living to 100 in the world's Blue Zones. As we were investigating these questions, I'd come home and be struck by how differently most Americans ate and lived compared to the Blue Zones residents I was visiting.

So my next step was to figure out how to bring those solutions back home. A major part of the quest was to research the foods and food practices common to all the Blue Zones, asking what we in America could learn from the food choices, recipes, menus, and ways of eating of the world's centenarians. What could we bring back and adapt to the kitchens, dining tables, and households of people here at home? I knew that it's one thing to know how to eat the right foods, but another to turn that into action. What could we do to get Americans back on track? People in the Blue Zones didn't struggle against their environments to be healthy; their surroundings actually drove healthy eating. Why were things so different here in the United States? That's when our team started a bold new experiment we called the Blue Zones Project, finding communities willing to make big changes to their environments to help people live longer and happier lives.

As it happened, that project had come to Fagen's hometown of Spencer a few months before he got his troubling diagnosis. Located at the fork of the Little Sioux and Ocheyedan Rivers in northwestern Iowa, Spencer has a Mayberry-esque Main Street, lined by quaint brick buildings and two Lutheran churches. Every September the Clay County Fair attracts 300,000 people, mostly rural Iowans, to inspect cattle, play games of chance, spin on rides, and eat deep-fried s'mores on a stick. A huge factory at the edge of town blends sugar, flavorings, and rendered pig cartilage to produce much of the nation's Jell-O. And in 1999 a Walmart sprang up about a mile outside of town. Now it attracts shoppers from dozens of small communities within a 50-mile radius to stock up on bargains, grab lunch at the Quiznos, Taco Bell, or Arby's, and drive home before dinner.

Spencer community leaders had invited us to present a plan to make permanent changes in the town to its living environment—changes based on the food preferences and cultural practices of the world's longest-lived people. Even though Spencer was a small town, home to only 11,193 people, residents here, like so many other Americans, were feeling increasingly isolated from one another. The Blue Zones Project offered them promise and gave them new opportunities to connect with others who wanted to live in a healthier community.

PROOF THAT IT WORKS

A compact man who favors bright polo shirts and often sports Oakley sunglasses, Bob Fagen has a slanty, conspiratorial smile that makes you feel like you're listening to the coolest kid in town. But on a blustery evening in November 2012, Fagen wasn't looking so cocky. As he took the podium in the ballroom of Spencer's Clay County Event Center, he shuffled his notes nervously. He looked out into the audience of 450 or so friends and neighbors, an audience that included some of the Blue Zones team members who had been working in Spencer that year. Many of us were still wearing parkas, having just come in from the whistling cold.

Fagen adjusted the microphone and leaned in. "Good evening," he said, pausing for a response that didn't come. "A year ago we invited the Blue Zones Project into our community, and it has begun to transform us." He went on to talk about all the changes that had happened so far. He described how he was leading the charge to rethink Main Street as a place not just for cars but also for humans. He mentioned new policies proposed by the city council to limit sprawl, to favor access to drinking water in public buildings, to ensure that everyone has easy, affordable access to vegetables, and to give everyone access to the gyms and playgrounds when school is out. He noted that the local Hy-Vee grocery store had started offering classes on cooking healthy, delicious meals. So far, he continued, about 750 people had signed a pledge to join the Blue Zones movement. Polite applause followed as he ticked off each accomplishment.

"Now I want to tell you a personal story," he said, shifting gears and raising his head earnestly. "Eight months ago, I discovered I had about a third of my kidney function left." The audience grew quiet. People shifted in their chairs. Fagen was a descendant of German farmers—stoic men who endured personal struggles privately. This was a different guy from the one the audience knew. Fagen told the story of his kidney failure, how his dad died, and the bargain he'd made with the specialist. "I wasn't going to die the same way," he proclaimed.

He began to walk more, in keeping with the Blue Zones theme of "moving naturally," he said. He also started eating better, including more salads. "Every time I sat down for a meal, I thought about Marybelle and Violet, my two granddaughters," he said. "I couldn't imagine not being there for them." Slowly but surely, he started feeling better.

"Well, I went back to see the specialist this week to get my latest tests and he gave me the news. My cholesterol and blood pressure are back to normal." Pausing with seemingly perfect, unpracticed timing, he delivered the punch line: "My kidneys are functioning at 100 percent."

Someone in the middle of the ballroom clapped, which set off a ripple, then a tsunami. Soon everyone was standing, applauding thunderously. Bob stepped back from the podium speechless, his face flushing red. The applause continued for several long moments and then ebbed. People sat down.

Fagen went back up to the microphone and pointed right at me, sitting in the front row with a few of my teammates. "These guys made a big difference in my life," he said. He was riding a bike, eating healthier foods, and spending more time with his family. He'd even run a 5K race. "I want you to give them a nice round of applause."

Because of the changes he had made in his life, Fagen was confident now that he'd live long enough to see Marybelle and Violet grow up, graduate from college, and walk down the aisle some day. "So I challenge all of you tonight," he said, tears welling in his eyes. "Think of whatever it is that's important to you. Don't wake up one day and wonder what happened to your life."

The audience was silent for a moment, then erupted again in applause.

Now I'm not an emotional guy, but I could feel my eyes welling up too—and not just at Fagen's story. For the past week I'd been visiting a series of Iowa towns that had signed up to become Blue Zones demonstration sites. In Waterloo, Cedar Falls, Mason City, and Spencer, I'd met with mayors, city managers, chamber of commerce presidents, superintendents of schools, and members of the local media. In each community as many as 40 percent of the adult population had pledged to follow our advice, starting with small adjustments to their eating habits, a gradual bump in physical activity, a weekly meeting with new friends—letting change radiate out through their lives and communities. We'd persuaded them all to align behind the idea of optimizing their towns for longevity and told them that, if we were successful, this could be the solution to reversing a living environment that had made 68 percent of Iowans overweight or obese. And they believed the message.

In my heart of hearts, I believed in the Blue Zones solutions. But I'm a guy who wants to see the numbers, and, when you put it that way, I didn't really know for sure. This was not a proven program; it was an experiment. I had researched the approach for years, and I knew variations of it had led to extraordinary longevity elsewhere around the world, but I wasn't sure it would work in Iowa, the epitome of Middle America. I felt like a guy way out over his skis with the ground approaching fast.

Until I heard Bob Fagen, that is. At that moment, for the first time, I realized that this idea was going to work. I caught my balance. Maybe we were really on to something.

SECRETS OF LIVING LONG

To tell the full story behind the life-changing ideas and practical, everyday advice I want to share with you in this book, I need to go back to the beginning. For more than a decade I've been working with the National Geographic Society to identify hot spots of longevity around the world—areas we called Blue Zones because a team of researchers had once circled a target region on a map with blue ink. Teaming up with demographer Michel Poulain, I set out to find the world's longest-lived people. We wanted to locate places that had not only high concentrations of 100-year-olds but also clusters of people who had grown old without diseases like heart problems, obesity, cancer, or diabetes. Poulain did extensive data analysis and research and pinpointed several regions in the world that appeared to have long-lived people. We needed to visit them to check birth and death records to confirm that these individuals were really as old as they thought they were. (In many places, the oldest individuals often don't know their ages, or might be lying about their ages, as was famously the case in Soviet Georgia in the 1970s.)

By 2009 we had found five places that met our criteria:

- **IKARIA, GREECE** An island in the Aegean Sea eight miles off the coast of Turkey that has one of the world's lowest rates of middle-age mortality and the lowest rates of dementia
- **OKINAWA, JAPAN** The largest island in a subtropical archipelago, home to the world's longest-lived women
- **OGLIASTRA REGION, SARDINIA** The mountainous highlands of an Italian island that boast the world's highest concentration of centenarian men
- **LOMA LINDA, CALIFORNIA** A community with the highest concentration of Seventh-day Adventists in the United States, where some residents live ten more healthy years than the average American
- **NICOYA PENINSULA, COSTA RICA** A place in this Central American country where residents have the world's lowest rates of middle-age mortality and the second highest concentration of male centenarians

To tease out the factors that contributed to longevity in these places, we assembled a team of leading medical researchers, anthropologists, dietitians, demographers, and epidemiologists. Piece by piece, we put together our working theories, collaborating with local researchers who were studying centenarians, cross-checking with academic papers, and interviewing a representative sample of 90- and 100-year-olds in each Blue Zone.

I found it especially helpful during my 20 or so trips to the Blue Zones to spend time just sitting with 100-year-olds and listening to their stories and paying attention to their lives. I watched as they prepared their meals, and I ate when and what they were used to eating. I knew that these people were doing something right—it wasn't just that they had won the genetic lottery. But what was it?

Remarkably, no matter where I found long-lived populations, I found similar habits and practices at work. When we asked our team of experts to identify these common denominators, they came up with these nine lessons, which we call the **Power Nine:**

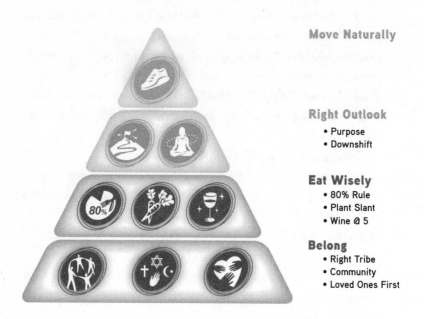

1. **Move Naturally.** The world's longest-lived people don't pump iron, run marathons, or join gyms. Instead, they live in environments that constantly nudge them into moving. They grow gardens and don't have mechanical conveniences for house and yard work. Every trip to work, to a friend's house, or to church occasions a walk.

2. **Purpose.** The Okinawans call it *ikigai* and the Nicoyans call it *plan de vida;* for both it translates to "why I wake up in the morning." In all Blue Zones people had something to live for beyond just work. Research has shown that knowing your sense of purpose is worth up to seven years of extra life expectancy.

3. **Downshift.** Even people in the Blue Zones experience stress, which leads to chronic inflammation, associated with every major age-related disease. The world's longest-lived people have routines

to shed that stress: Okinawans take a few moments each day to remember their ancestors, Adventists pray, Ikarians take a nap, and Sardinians do happy hour.

4. **80 Percent Rule.** *Hara hachi bu*—the 2,500-year-old Confucian mantra spoken before meals on Okinawa—reminds people to stop eating when their stomachs are 80 percent full. The 20 percent gap between not being hungry and feeling full could be the difference between losing weight and gaining it. People in the Blue Zones eat their smallest meal in the late afternoon or early evening, and then they don't eat any more the rest of the day.

5. **Plant Slant.** Beans, including fava, black, soy, and lentil, are the cornerstone of most centenarian diets. Meat—mostly pork—is eaten on average only five times per month, and in a serving of three to four ounces, about the size of a deck of cards.

6. **Wine @ 5.** People in all Blue Zones (even some Adventists) drink alcohol moderately and regularly. Moderate drinkers outlive nondrinkers. The trick is to drink one to two glasses per day with friends and/or with food. And no, you can't save up all week and have 14 drinks on Saturday.

7. **Right Tribe.** The world's longest-lived people choose, or were born into, social circles that support healthy behaviors. Okinawans create *moais*—groups of five friends that commit to each other for life. Research shows that smoking, obesity, happiness, and even loneliness are contagious. By contrast, social networks of long-lived people favorably shape their health behaviors.

8. **Community.** All but 5 of the 263 centenarians we interviewed belonged to a faith-based community. Denomination doesn't seem to matter. Research shows that attending faith-based services four times per month will add 4 to 14 years of life expectancy.

9. **Loved Ones First.** Successful centenarians in the Blue Zones put their families first. They keep aging parents and grandparents nearby or in the home, which also lowers disease and mortality rates of their children. They commit to a life partner (which can add up to three years of life expectancy), and they invest in their

children with time and love, which makes the children more likely to be caretakers when the time comes.

What we discovered in every Blue Zone, as the Power Nine suggest, is that the path to a long, healthy life comes from creating an environment around yourself, your family, and your community that nudges you into following the right behaviors subtly and relentlessly, just as the Blue Zones do for their populations.

COULD I BLUE ZONE AMERICA?

After my first book, *The Blue Zones,* made the *New York Times* best sellers list, I was invited onto television shows—*Good Morning America, Oprah, Today, Headline News, Fox and Friends,* and on CNN with Sanjay Gupta—several dozen talk shows in all. But even when the Blue Zones were in the headlines, I knew that right behind me there would be another health expert sitting in the same interview seat the next day, promoting another idea, another diet, another way to get healthy.

I didn't want what we'd learned in the Blue Zones to be dismissed like yesterday's fad. We'd used science to unearth some profound secrets from people around the world who lived long, happy, healthy lives, and now I could sense a bigger purpose for all the research we'd been doing if I could use all we had discovered to help Americans get healthier. I could tell that they craved this kind of information. I knew we were onto something more encompassing than another diet plan. Eating habits were central, but they weren't the whole picture. All the research showed that diets didn't work, but the Blue Zones lifestyle did. To follow the Blue Zones approach meant making changes in lifestyle and environment, not just daily menus. If these ideas were broadcast out to an even bigger sphere, what might happen? I began to wonder if a community could decide to become a Blue Zone—could turn itself around and become healthier by following habits like those in the Blue Zones, places where better lifestyle habits had evolved over time. Had anyone ever managed to successfully manufacture a new Blue Zone?

I began digging into the medical health literature, looking for examples, and I found exactly one: a bold experiment in an obscure region in northern Europe that had produced miraculous results during the 1970s. Back then, the North Karelia region of Finland was home to the world's unhealthiest population by several measures. But an innovative group of young scientists and public health virtuosos, led by an amazing fellow named Pekka Puska, had developed a grassroots strategy and made broad-reaching changes in the food and eating habits—and in the health and well-being—of the North Karelians. Those changes reduced heart disease by 80 percent and cancer by 60 percent among the 170,000 working-age people there. After reading about the project and then corresponding for a while with Puska, I went to see for myself. I had to learn how this team of determined people managed to change the health profile of an entire community.

Could the same thing be done here in the United States? We were in the midst of a health crisis. If current trends continued, three-fourths of us would be overweight or obese and half of us would be suffering from diabetes by 2030. The average American was already lugging a fifth more body fat (the equivalent of three gallons or so of flab) than in 1970. But it didn't have to be that way. Our research suggested that if Americans could follow the examples of people in the Blue Zones, we could all lose an average of 20 pounds. We would suffer about half the rate of heart disease and about a fifth the rate of diabetes and certain cancers. We'd enjoy an average of eight more good years than we do now. But how could we make that happen?

A NEW PATHWAY TO HEALTH

If we want to improve the health and lifestyle of Americans, maybe we've been going about it the wrong way, I thought. Maybe we need to expand our focus from individual diet and exercise regimens all the way out to entire communities and what they offer to help people make changes. Maybe we need to reshape whole towns if we wanted to add healthy years to the people living in them. I started to get excited about the idea of weaving Blue Zones principles into the fabric of a community—from the food on breakfast tables to the lunches served in school cafeterias, from one person's exercise regimen to bike lanes on downtown streets—so that residents of all ages would be constantly nudged into making healthier choices without even thinking about it. After all, they'd done something similar in northern Finland. Why couldn't we do it too?

When I started looking for communities in the United States that were already thinking along these lines, I realized that American cities span the range of how "blue" they are. Some have high Blue Zones–style ratings, like San Luis Obispo, California, and Charlottesville, Virginia, where less than 15 percent of the residents are obese. Others are more like Binghamton, New York, or Huntington, West Virginia, where about 38 percent of the residents are seriously overweight. Is that because people in San Luis Obispo and Charlottesville have better genes than those in Binghamton and Huntington, or because they have a greater desire to see their families be healthy? No. It's because of the culture of these communities, supported by conscientious leaders committed to creating a healthier environment for their citizens. It's easier for people in those towns to stay healthy because they live in a place that supports them rather than constantly undermines them.

I began my research by consulting public health experts in my home state, at the University of Minnesota. They told me that I should rigorously measure any campaign we organized so that we could assess how well it was working, and they warned me to be very careful about what we recommended, because people's lives would be affected. And it wouldn't be cheap, we discovered. At a minimum, a community-wide initiative like the one we envisioned—even one with a strong grassroots base—could cost a million dollars. Where would we get that kind of money? The National Institutes of Health, I learned, had funded similar "heart healthy" campaigns during the 1980s, but none had successfully proved that their multimillion-dollar budgets would result in major health improvements. How was I going to get the money for the Blue Zones Project if the country's best experts had failed?

As it turned out, executives at AARP had also been thinking about organizing a community-wide health initiative. When I told them about my strategy to focus on environment instead of individual behavior change as a way to nudge people into eating better and living longer, they rallied behind me. In 2009, with the backing of the University of Minnesota School of Public Health, AARP provided me funds for a pilot project. Since then, the Blue Zones Project has worked with 20 different communities, learning every step of the way how to use the indigenous wisdom of the world's centenarians to bring health and longevity into our own lives. As a result of our efforts, more than five million people today live in communities that support better health behaviors. Most of those five million have made life-enhancing changes without ever having to think about it. In some cities, we've seen a reduction in obesity of greater than 10 percent coupled with a reduction of smoking of 30 percent.

EATING THE BLUE ZONES WAY

You might be reading this now and saying, *All these stories about the Blue Zones are fine, but I don't live on an island in the Mediterranean, and you haven't come to my hometown yet.* Or you might be saying, *I live in a town where fast-food restaurants abound, and I'm busy with family and work and trying to stay on a budget. Grocery store vegetables often look limp and are still expensive. Stores that carry plenty of good, healthy food are few and far away. It's much easier and cheaper to stop at the burger or pizza restaurant.* You might be saying, *I live in a place built for cars. I drive to work, to the store, to my place of worship; things are spread out. There's stress-inducing and sometimes dangerous traffic. My friends are busy, too, and they live a long way from me. I don't have time to get together for dinner. How can I be expected to eat and live like people in the Blue Zones? It's not realistic. No way I can do in my life what Bob Fagen did in his to get healthier.*

I understand. Across the nation, there are still so many Americans who deserve to enjoy the same benefits as the communities in our Blue Zones Project. In so many parts of the country, Americans are still drowning in a sea of cheap calories that are impossible to escape. We can't walk through an airport, pay cash for gasoline, or buy cough medicine without being confronted by a barrage of salty snacks, candy bars, and sodas. High-sugar snacks are even disguised as "health bars." Restaurateurs have figured out that they can make a bigger profit with bigger servings. So often we overeat when we go out for breakfast, lunch, or dinner. With help from the brightest minds on Madison Avenue, the food industry spends $11 billion a year to entice us to buy their products—mostly sugared, salted, flavor-enhanced processed foods like pizzas, pastries, chips, and sodas. The average American now consumes 46 slices of pizza, 200 pounds of meat, and 607 pounds of milk and other dairy products, and washes it down with 57 gallons of soda pop a year. We consume 8,000 teaspoons of added sugar and 79 pounds of fat annually. We eat 4.5 billion pounds of fries and 2 billion pounds of chips a year.

Does that mean we're bad people? That we lack the discipline of our forefathers? That we care less about our health and our children's health than our grandparents did? Of course not. Then what has happened in this past half century? We've gone from an environment of hardship and scarcity to one of abundance and ease. How can we make the most of this abundance without letting it ruin our health?

The traditional answer has always had something to do with individual responsibility: Get on a diet and exercise program! The problem with that plan is that it requires long-term discipline and routine—both of which go against human nature and our evolutionary design. The human psyche craves the new and the novel; we get bored. Even if a strategy works for a while, the urge to try something new eventually takes over. Most people stick with diets for less than seven months, and often only weeks. Of 100 people who start a diet today, fewer than 5 will still be on that diet's maintenance plan two years later. As a strategy to lose weight—much less to avoid heart attacks or live longer—diets are largely useless. Deploying discipline is like using a muscle. At a certain point, muscles fatigue, and eventually we break down and eat that bag of potato chips.

The Blue Zones Solution offers an alternative—food ideas and eating practices, plus ways to change your environment that make it all the more likely that you will live a longer, healthier life. We've adapted the lessons from the original Blue Zones, piloted the lifestyle changes in real communities, and translated the actual foods into easy, doable recipes designed for every taste and family—kids included—and die-hard meat-and-potato lovers too. We want you to love what you eat, how you spend your day, and the people around you. We want you to feel your life is getting better and better, whether you start by embracing the Blue Zones Solution on a small scale at home or are inspired to get involved in transforming your whole neighborhood, extended family, town, or city.

FORGET TO DIE

You can ask centenarians what they've done to make it to 100, as I have many times, but few of them really know. Some say it was the wine they drank or the clean air they breathed; others will say it was the daily walks they took or even the daily cigars they enjoyed. I once pressed a 101-year-old woman living in Ikaria, Greece, to tell me why she thought people there lived so long. "We just forget to die," she said with a shrug. Actually she was more right than she knew. None of the 253 spry centenarians I've met went on a diet, joined a gym, or took supplements. They didn't pursue longevity—it simply ensued.

As a burgeoning body of research has suggested, we, too, can make long-term changes to our personal environment that will nudge us into moving more, socializing more, hungering for less, and eating better. In other words, we can make decisions right now that will lead to a healthier, happier future.

This book is about making sure that vitality *ensues* for you. In part 1 you'll travel with me and share meals with remarkable people in all five Blue Zones, and you'll learn what our subsequent research has told us about the foods they eat and the role of eating in their lives. In part 2 you'll read about a few of our recent Blue Zones city makeovers, learning how each community finds its own path to health and longevity, following the lead of the world's centenarians. I hope this will help you see that change is possible no matter where you live or how you and your family now eat, and perhaps inspire you to get involved in transforming your own community.

In part 3 you'll find a wealth of information and step-by-step guidelines on creating your own Blue Zone, and in part 4 you'll find 77 recipes. Some come from my centenarian friends in the Blue Zones around the world and have been adapted for American kitchens. Others come from my kitchen, from my friends at home and in makeover cities, and from some of the country's top chefs, many of whom already understand the value of cooking and eating the Blue Zones way.

My ultimate goal in writing this book—besides sharing with you the best Blue Zones foods as well as delicious ways to prepare them and powerful practices to enjoy them with your family and friends—is for you to have a Bob Fagen moment of your own: When you discover that, without knowing exactly how or when it happened, you're healthier and happier than you ever thought possible.

PART ONE

Discovering the Blue Zones

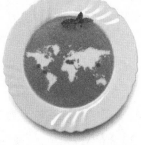

I T WAS A MEAL TO REMEMBER. We were sitting at a table overlooking the Aegean Sea on the Greek island of Ikaria. Spread before us were plates of fresh fish, black-eyed peas with fennel, Greek salad, sourdough bread, and local wine—food that radiated health. I couldn't have been happier.

My lunch companion was Antonia Trichopoulou of the University of Athens, the world's leading expert on the Mediterranean diet. Thinking of all the research she'd done, I asked her how I could persuade Americans to start eating food as healthy as this. I expected her to tell me I should focus on the dozens of nutritional benefits of the Ikarian diet. Instead, she motioned to the delicious items before us and said, "Feed them!"

It was Trichopoulou's insight that gave me the organizing principle for this book. No one thing explains longevity in the Blue Zones. It's really an interconnected web of factors—including what we eat, our social network, daily rituals, physical environment, and sense of purpose—that propels us forward and gives life meaning. But food is at the center of that ecosystem, and food may be the best starting point for anyone seeking to emulate the health, longevity, and well-being found in the world's Blue Zones.

We make decisions about what to eat several times each day. Apart from the obvious health ramifications, these decisions also determine how we spend our time. Do we shed stress by growing food in a garden? Do we prepare meals with our family? Do we unwind with conversation over a good meal? Or do we grab a bite on the run at a drive-through so we can cram more activity into our already busy days?

Food also helps determine the company we keep and how we keep our company. If you invite a vegetarian friend over for dinner, you'll probably make an effort to prepare a healthy salad and a creative, meatless main dish. By contrast, if your friend's idea of a balanced meal is a burger in each hand, you'll probably find yourself eating a big, greasy burger too.

For many of us, food choices flow from our belief systems, dictating whether we eat fish on Friday, challah at sundown, unleavened bread on the Sabbath, or no food at all during certain times of the year. Every time we take a bite, we vote for the world we want to inhabit: Are we supporting a system that favors a healthy climate and environment or are we helping to pollute our surroundings? Are we buying foods produced by our neighbors or foods made in factories from ingredients we hardly recognize? If we choose not to eat meat, are we doing it because of nutritional or ethical concerns?

For all of these reasons, food is the perfect runway to a Blue Zones approach to a longer, healthier life. In this first part of the book, we'll explore five of the world's Blue Zones through the lens of food. You'll see the eating choices and practices of centenarians in each location along with fascinating research about their diets and dining habits, as determined by dozens of dietary surveys and studies during the past century or so. By the time we're done, I think you'll see that the secret to eating to 100 lies not only in what the centenarians ate but, more important, how food fit into their lives—not just the nutritional value of ingredients but also where food is grown, how it's prepared, what rituals surround it, when it's consumed, and with whom. My guess is that, once you know what it's like to eat in a Blue Zone, you too will be hungry for the same kind of food—and for the same kind of lifestyle that surrounds it.

CHAPTER ONE

❧

The Secrets of a Mediterranean Diet: Ikaria, Greece

L ATE ONE SUMMER AFTERNOON I sat perched on a counter stool in the kitchen of Thea Parikos's guesthouse on the Greek island of Ikaria. The guesthouse sits on a rise, overlooking a cobalt blue stretch of the Aegean Sea. Faintly visible in the distance is the thin hazy line of Turkey's western coast.

At the top of the hill behind the guesthouse, past prickly scrub, rocky riverbeds, and unlikely vegetable gardens, lies the mountain village of Christos Raches. Here, in small homesteads shadowed by cedar forests, reside some of the world's longest-lived people—people who live eight years longer than Americans typically do, with half the rate of heart disease and almost no dementia. The people of Ikaria have what the rest of us want: long, healthy lives with vitality until the very end.

I've made regular research visits to Ikaria during the past few years and enjoyed many meals at the guesthouse. But this was the first time I'd been invited inside the guesthouse kitchen.

As I looked around the warrenlike space, dimly lit by two small windows, I saw a jumble of warped pans and dented pots hanging from the wall. A snarl of just harvested vegetables and foraged greens blanketed the counter opposite me. Above them, great shrubberies of dried oregano, sage, and thyme descended from the ceiling like chandeliers. On the tanklike industrial stove, a pressure cooker whistled steam while smaller pots bubbled with ingredients like black-eyed peas, parsley, feral chicken, feta goat cheese, eggplant, wild asparagus, and fennel. The aromas from the stove were intoxicating: herbal, meaty, deliciously musky, and—I can think of no other adjective—fecund.

At the center of this holy chaos stood Athina Mazari, a 58-year-old master of Ikarian cuisine. In a controlled frenzy, she moved swiftly from task to task, using only the simplest of culinary tools, chopping, mixing, stirring, tasting, and then correcting ingredients. Almost everything that went into Mazari's dishes came from the nearby gardens that spilled down the mountainside. It struck me as I watched her that I was witnessing one of the world's great workshops of longevity.

I'd been nagging Mazari for years to let me watch her do her magic in the kitchen. But she'd always made it clear that she would rather prepare food alone, enjoying the wordless routine of her work. Today, for some reason, she made an exception. After all this time, I guess I'd worn her down. Between cooking tasks, she opened up.

Her journey to the guesthouse kitchen had been a long one. Like most Ikarian children of the 1950s, she was born into a large family and hardship. Neither she nor her eight siblings had received more than an elementary education. While her brothers helped their father in the fields, Mazari and her sisters apprenticed in the kitchen, chopping vegetables and washing dishes. There she began to absorb the island's traditional cooking wisdom, combining the same few dozen ingredients and preparing them in the same way as her ancestors have done since the sixth century B.C.

"I made my first loaf of bread when I was ten," she said. It was sourdough bread. "I borrowed the starter dough from a neighbor." Kneading it with rye flour, salt, and water, she waited for it to rise overnight and then baked it in the wood-fired brick oven behind her house. The bacteria that fermented the bread came from the same starter culture that her neighbor's great-great-grandmother had used.

One day Mazari's mother called her into the kitchen. She said the family was no longer able to make ends meet. Mazari would be moving in with a young couple in the village that had just had a baby and needed a nanny. In exchange for room and board, she would cook, clean, and take care of the newborn child. She'd learn the skills she'd need herself when she became a mother one day. Mazari was nine years old.

Over the next decade Mazari would be a nanny for three different families. Each time, as she cooked alongside the woman of the house, she acquired more kitchen skills and picked up more recipes. She learned how to cube and steam vegetables according to size and texture so they all delivered the right crunch; to poke a pork roast to discern how well done it was; to measure ingredients by hand, literally; to roll dried oregano between her palms and scatter it perfectly with an operatic wave; to instantly recognize by smell the freshness of fish.

She knew where the island's 80 or so varieties of wild greens—*horta*—grew, in which months to pick them, and how to bake them into savory pies. She learned how to dry surplus vegetables on the roof, hanging them in mesh bags for storage. Then, as summer turned to winter, her meals changed from fresh vegetables and fish to pork-seasoned stews, root vegetables, and winter cabbage soup. Her culinary repertoire grew to more than a hundred recipes—all in her head, all assembled and prepared by feel and driven by epicurean instinct.

In her 20s, Mazari grew into a great beauty. She recalled how men would stop and stare as she walked by, and one of those men caught her eye. Soon they were married, and in a few years she had two children of her own to cook for. And although her children were now all grown up, she was still cooking for others.

As Mazari's story unfolded and her dishes neared completion, I sat on my stool in awe. She had talked nonstop, but it hadn't interfered with her effortless orchestration of tasks. I wondered if the treadmill of preparing fabulous meals three times daily for almost a half century, only to have them end in a pile of dirty dishes to wash, had taken the enjoyment out of her cooking.

Mazari suddenly stopped what she was doing and fixed me with a long look. "When I was in my late 30s, we were short of money, and I worked for a while as chambermaid in a small hotel near my village," she said. "One day the chef didn't show up and the hotel owner, a woman named

Maria, asked if I could step in. Twenty-six American artists had shown up for dinner and she wanted to know if I could cook. She let me set the menu, and I prepared pies made from wild greens, stuffed grapevine leaves with rice, Greek salad with *tzatziki* dressing. When I put all the food out on plates, I realized it didn't look like restaurant food I'd seen in pictures. When Maria came into the kitchen to serve the food, I said to her, 'I'm sorry these don't look nice, but they taste nice.' I was very nervous."

It was now late afternoon in the guesthouse kitchen. The soft sun suffused the room in a medieval light. Mazari leaned against the opposing counter and rubbed her coarse, damp hands, as she remembered that moment long ago.

"Maria suddenly shouted for me from the dining room," she said. "I thought she was mad at me—that I had embarrassed her, and that I needed to do the dishes over. Instead, when I walked out of the kitchen, all of the foreigners stood up and gave me a standing ovation. My eyes welled up with tears. I tried to hold them back but I couldn't. It was the first time in my life I cried with joy."

THE BEST MEDITERRANEAN DIET

Almost every mother and grandmother on the island possesses a culinary pedigree like Mazari's, I've found. Like other Blue Zones, Ikaria is remote, and people have stuck to their traditions, which have enabled them to avoid the influence of modern Western eating habits. Their tradition of preparing the right foods, in the right way, I believe, has a lot to do with the island's longevity.

Our research backs this up. During one of our team's visits to Ikaria, we worked with Trichopoulou, the authority on the Mediterranean diet, to administer surveys of local eating habits. As data from the surveys started coming in, Trichopoulou noted that the island's traditional diet, like that found in much of the Mediterranean, included lots of vegetables and olive oil, smaller amounts of dairy and meat products, and moderate amounts of alcohol. What set it apart from other places in the region was its emphasis on potatoes, goat's milk, honey, legumes (especially garbanzo beans, black-eyed peas, and lentils), wild greens, some fruit, and relatively small amounts of fish.

Every one of these foods has been linked to increased longevity. Low dairy consumption has been associated with reduced heart disease. Olive oil—especially unheated—is believed to lower bad cholesterol and increase good cholesterol. Goat's milk contains serotonin-boosting tryptophan. Some wild greens contain ten times as many antioxidants as red wine. And wine—in moderation—has been shown to be beneficial if consumed as part of a Mediterranean diet, because it helps the body absorb more of the flavonoids, the artery-scrubbing antioxidants, from the food eaten with it.

Even coffee, the habit your grandmother once warned you about, has been linked to lower rates of diabetes, heart disease, and, for some, Parkinson's disease. Local sourdough bread contains *Lactobacillus sanfranciscensis,* a health-boosting type of bacteria that, when eaten with other food, may actually reduce the meal's glycemic index. (A food's glycemic index reflects how fast it breaks down to sugar in the bloodstream. Meals with a lower glycemic index will take longer to digest and are less likely to cause a spike in blood sugar levels.) Potatoes have heart-healthy potassium, vitamin B_6, and fiber. And, as Trichopoulou observed during our research trip, islanders inevitably consume fewer chemicals because they eat greens from their own gardens or nearby fields. Considering all this, she told me, compared to the standard American diet, the Ikarian diet may add up to four years to the life expectancy of islanders.

We gained more insight into traditional island foods from Ioannna Chinou, a leading authority on the bioactive properties of herbs and other natural foods. She pointed out that different Greek teas may offer specific beneficial effects: wild mint as a way to prevent gingivitis and ulcers, rosemary to treat gout, artemisia to improve blood circulation. When I brought her samples of Ikarian herbal teas to test in her lab, Chinou found that they all had antioxidant properties. In addition, the teas appeared to function as mild diuretics, helping to flush waste products from the body and slightly lower blood pressure.

Five years after I began looking into the healthy habits of Ikarians, a Greek researcher named Christina Chrysohoou published the first academic paper on the Ikarian diet. By day Chrysohoou sees patients as a cardiologist at the University of Athens School of Medicine. By night she somehow finds the energy to follow her wide-ranging intellectual interests.

Chrysohoou was the first academic to recognize the scientific potential of Ikaria as a study site to examine how psychology, depression, obesity, and even radiation might influence longevity. In 2009 she and Demosthenes B. Panagiotakos of Harokopio University organized *The Ikaria Study* that surveyed 1,420 Ikarians, testing 673 of them over age 65. Amazingly, 79 of them were over age 90. Their research teams fanned out across the island, collecting more than 300 pieces of information on each subject, mostly on diet but also detailed medical histories, including information about sleep, depression, and even sex habits. Four years later, the team returned to Ikaria to check up on their oldest subjects.

The team confirmed that Ikarians have followed an extreme and unique version of the Mediterranean diet, which favors vegetables, whole grains, fruits, fish, olive oil, goat's milk and cheese, and wine. The researchers observed that fresh vegetables are always in season on Ikaria: potatoes and onions in the fall, cabbage in the winter, and lettuce in the spring. Summer brings peppers, green beans, tomatoes, zucchini, eggplants, apricots, and peaches: These foods the islanders eat fresh or sun-dried and preserved with oregano for winter. Wild greens such as dandelion, chicory, and wild fennel abound, providing a rich source of vitamins A, C, and K, folate, potassium, magnesium, calcium, fiber, and iron. While fat accounts for more than 50 percent of their daily calories, more than half the fat energy comes from olive oil, associated with positive health factors in a number of studies.

Islanders eat relatively more legumes (especially garbanzos, lentils, and black-eyed peas), potatoes, coffee, herbal teas, and wild greens than do people in other Mediterranean cultures. Perhaps due to the island's famously rough seas, Ikarians traditionally have eaten fish only sporadically, as fishermen have been able to get out. While coastal dwellers enjoy swordfish, sardines, anchovies, and small local fish varieties six to eight times per month, mountain dwellers eat fish only once or

Typical Daily Diet of Ikarians Age 80-Plus
(Percentage of daily intake in grams)

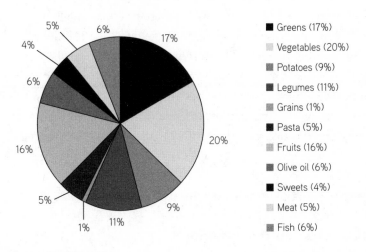

- Greens (17%)
- Vegetables (20%)
- Potatoes (9%)
- Legumes (11%)
- Grains (1%)
- Pasta (5%)
- Fruits (16%)
- Olive oil (6%)
- Sweets (4%)
- Meat (5%)
- Fish (6%)

Source: Chrysohoou [1].

Older Ikarians eat a diet rich in greens and other vegetables, beans, and fruit, which together account for 64 percent of their daily food intake—dairy products and beverages excluded. Fat accounts for more than 50 percent of their daily calories, but more than half the fat energy comes from olive oil, associated with positive health factors in a number of studies.

twice a month, and often partially preserved fish such as salted cod or sardines. Interestingly, we found more healthy islanders age 90-plus in the mountains than on the coast, so fish doesn't seem to be contributing to longevity. Ikarians typically consume meat only once or twice a week, poultry twice a week, and sweets perhaps twice a week, not counting the local honey they use to sweeten their tea.

Chrysohoou identified several nonfood habits that she believes also contribute to the longevity of islanders. For instance, Ikarians tend to eat slowly and with families or friends. They also take regular naps. In fact, a 2008 paper by the University of Athens Medical School and the Harvard School of Public Health reported findings after following a group of Greeks over several decades. The researchers found that regular napping—at least five days weekly—decreased a person's risk of heart disease by 37 percent.

Ikarians tend to have other ways they unwind, Chrysohoou has found. She showed me a preliminary study suggesting that roughly 80 percent of Ikarian males between the ages of 65 and 85 were still having sex. "This means less stress, and that means healthier eating," she speculated. "When you eat a meal in a hurry or with pent-up worry, stress hormones like cortisol interfere with the digestive process. Your body doesn't absorb nutrients and antioxidants as well; the calories you consume are more likely to end up as fat on your waistline than energy for your cells."

TOP LONGEVITY FOODS FROM IKARIA

Ikarian cooks, like their counterparts in places such as France, Spain, or Italy, lean heavily on dishes that include vegetables, whole grains, fruits, olive oil, and occasionally a little fish.

OLIVE OIL In Greece the finest extra-virgin olive oil—extracted without any treatment other than washing the fruit, pressing, decanting, and filtration—tends to be cloudy, slightly thick, and a deep golden green. A fondness for the best olive oil may protect Ikarians from heart disease. A recent study in Spain found that a healthy low-fat Mediterranean diet that includes at least four tablespoons of olive oil a day—a typical amount for these Greek islanders—reduces the risk of heart disease by 30 percent. In Ikaria, we found that people consuming at least 100 grams (about four tablespoons, or a quarter cup) of good olive oil a day had 50 percent lower mortality.

WILD GREENS More than 150 varieties of wild greens, such as purslane, dandelion, and arugula, grow all over the island. These rich, dark, wild mountain greens are a great source of minerals like iron, magnesium, potassium, and calcium, as well as carotenoids—the colorful pigments the body converts to Vitamin A. Eating a cup of greens daily seemed to be one of the keys to a longer life in Ikaria. In North America we have plenty of edible wild greens—dandelion, purslane, lamb's-quarter—and cultivated greens such as collard, mustard greens, beet greens, and kale have nearly the same plenitude of nutrients.

POTATOES Unique among Mediterranean peoples, Ikarians eat potatoes almost daily. Despite high carbs, potatoes offer significant health benefits. Recent studies have suggested that, as long as they're not fried or loaded up with sour cream and butter, potatoes can help reduce blood pressure, prevent inflammation, and fight diabetes.

FETA CHEESE Bioactive Ikarian feta cheese is made by fermenting goat's milk with rennin, which the Ikarians get from goats' stomachs. The result is a protein-rich probiotic high in gut-friendly bacteria with powerful anti-inflammatory and anticancer properties. Famously added to Greek salads, feta is also used by the Ikarians to round out several vegetable stews and other dishes.

BLACK-EYED PEAS Called peas but actually beans, these Ikarian favorites are rich in protein and fiber. They have also been found to contain some of the strongest anticancer, anti-diabetes, and heart-protective substances in nature.

CHICKPEAS Included in many stews and soups, chickpeas are also eaten like a snack on Ikaria, dried and salted like peanuts. They are higher in fat than other beans, but nearly all of their fat is unsaturated, which makes them a healthy choice that avoids the sugar rush that higher-carbohydrate snacks might cause.

LEMONS Ikarians put lemon juice on everything. They eat the whole fruit, skin and all. The high acidity of lemon peels may have a beneficial impact on blood glucose, helping to control or prevent diabetes. Ikarians squeeze lemon on salads, fish, soups, and beans and into drinking water, lowering the glycemic load of the entire meal.

MEDITERRANEAN HERBS Drinking herbal tea is an island ritual. Garden and wild herbs make fragrant, seasonal, and healthful drinks. From rosemary they get a heady rush of rosmarinic acid, carnosic acid, and carnosol—substances that have been shown to protect against certain cancers in animal studies. Marjoram offers ursolic acid, which may boost memory and other cognitive functions. Daily teas made from sage, rosemary, marjoram, and mint—all containing diuretics and anti-inflammatories—may explain Ikaria's very low dementia rate. Adding ample culinary herbs, preferably fresh, to cooked dishes captures some of those nutrients as well.

COFFEE They like their coffee strong on Ikaria. Two to three cups a day of Turkish-style Ikarian coffee have been shown to reduce mortality rates for both men and women in recent studies.

HONEY Islanders use Ikarian honey—dark, thick, and rich—as a medicine to treat everything from colds and insomnia to healing wounds. Besides stirring it into coffee or tea, many older folks also take it neat, by the spoonful, first thing in the morning and again at night before dinner.

For recipes from Ikaria, see pages 244–255.

❧

CHAPTER TWO

A Diet From the World's Longest-Lived Women: Okinawa, Japan

I T TOOK ME TWO DAYS TO CONVINCE Gozei Shinzato to show me her arsenal of longevity supplements, but, in the end, she delivered.

Before me lay at least five compounds that could explain how the spry centenarian had eluded the diseases of aging to reach her 104th year with the flexibility of a yogi and the frenetic energy of a Chihuahua. She showed me one supercharged supplement with carotenoids, flavonoids, and saponins, and another that fights breast cancer by reducing blood estrogen. She pointed to a proven antimalarial agent that she uses to keep her stomach healthy, another that has been shown to help regulate metabolism, maintain low blood pressure, treat gallstones, and work as a prophylactic for hangovers. She reached down to pick up one that lowers blood sugar to help stave off diabetes. Three of them have proven antiaging properties.

While this may sound like the inventory of a well-stocked medicine cabinet, we were actually standing in Shinzato's kitchen garden. The "supplements" on display were Okinawan sweet potatoes, soybeans, mugwort, turmeric, and *goya* (bitter melon). All of these grew in neat rows, just 15 steps outside of her house.

The day before, I'd traveled to her village in northern Okinawa with two longevity experts, gerontologist Craig Willcox, who along with his brother Bradley wrote the *New York Times* best seller *The Okinawa Diet Plan*, and Greg Plotnikoff, a U.S.-trained physician and authority on integrative medicine. Both of these men supremely understand how food can work as medicine—or as poison. We spent the day interviewing Shinzato about her diet, observing her lifestyle, and watching her prepare a traditional Okinawan meal. We watched her spring up and down from her tatami mat more than a dozen times. We learned that Shinzato's life was one of comforting routine. She lived alone in a furniture-less, three-room house partitioned by rice-paper doors. Upon awaking, she wrapped her elfin 85-pound frame in a cobalt blue kimono. Then she made an offering at the ancestor shrine in her living room, lighting incense on a small altar cluttered with old photographs, a tortoiseshell comb, an urn, and other relics from her forebears.

Then, in the cool hours of the day, she worked in her garden. After lunch, she read comic books or watched a baseball game on television and napped. Neighbors stopped by every afternoon, and a couple of days a week her *moai*—four women who, together with Shinzato, had at a young age committed to one another for life—stopped by for mugwort tea and conversation. Whenever things had gotten rough in Shinzato's life, when she'd run short of cash or when her husband had died 46 years ago, she'd counted on her moai and the Okinawan sense of social obligation—*yuimaru*—to support her. Her friends had relied on a lifetime of Shinzato's support in return.

We watched her make jasmine tea, squatting in the corner and pouring hot water over tea leaves as the room filled with a delicate, floral aroma. At lunch, she mixed homemade miso into a saucepan of water. She spooned in fresh carrots, radishes, shiitake mushrooms, and tofu, and let it heat. Meanwhile, she moved up and down the kitchen wiping clean the counters, sink, and even the window. Then she pulled up a chair facing the stove to wait for her soup. The flame cast a feeble light on Shinzato's creased but serene face. She spiced the soup with a sauce of marinated garlic and herbs—"longevity medicines," Plotnikoff observed. Her movements were slow and careful with a patient, tortoise-like resolve; she seemed completely oblivious of us.

She poured her warmed soup into a bowl, gazed at it for a few long moments, and murmured, *"Hara hachi bu."* This Confucian adage, intoned like a prayer before every meal, reminded her to stop eating when she was 80 percent full. She threw me a quick glance and then looked back at the steaming bowl, seemingly waiting for something. Then I realized: Perhaps she wanted to eat in private? I announced that we had to leave. "Thank you very much," I said to her, bowing slightly. "May we come back and see your garden tomorrow?"

"If you must," she quipped, fixing me with her mirthful, pinched smile. Or was that a wince?

Rain fell lightly the following day when we returned to her house. It was a chilly gray morning. Willcox, Plotnikoff, and I stood towering over Shinzato, who measures about four and a half feet tall in platform thongs. Across the road, past a few peasant homes and a small stream, was rioting jungle—viper habitat—that blanketed a mountainside. Shinzato's garden glistened damply in luminescent shades of chartreuse and emerald. We asked Shinzato about her garden. What grows best? (Sweet potatoes.) Was there a longevity food? (No.) What do you use as fertilizer? (Fishmeal.) How many hours per day do you work in the garden? (Four.) What is your favorite part about gardening? (Solitude.) She endured our questions with polite serenity, rain dripping off of her wide, conical hat.

During a brief lull in our inquisition, she excused herself to dive back into her garden. Armed with a three-pronged hoe, Shinzato began attacking weeds. Working with a mechanical ferocity, she ripped at the red, rocky soil, working her way up and down the planted rows. Then, on a small rubber pad, she knelt down to pull small weeds by hand. We watched her for perhaps a half hour, taking pictures and making notes, until we got our fill. I walked over and tapped Shinzato on the shoulder and told her we were going. She looked up at me and tersely bid me farewell in Okinawan. I asked Willcox to translate.

"She said 'good,'" Willcox responded. "Though I'm not sure if she means it was good to meet us or it is good to see us go . . ."

THE RISE AND FALL OF A GREAT LONGEVITY DIET

Okinawa is sort of a Japanese Hawaii—an exotic, laid-back group of islands with warm weather, palm trees, and sugar-sand beaches. For almost a thousand years, this Pacific archipelago has maintained a reputation for nurturing extreme longevity. Okinawans over the age of 65 enjoy the world's highest life expectancy. The average life expectancy for men is 80, and for women it's about 88. Men are expected to live to about 84, while women are expected to live to almost age 90. People here also have one of the highest centenarian ratios: About 6.5 in 10,000 live to age 100. They suffer only a fraction of diseases that kill Americans: a fifth the rate of cardiovascular disease, a fifth the rate of breast and prostate cancer, and less than half the rate of dementia seen among similarly aged Americans.

What was Shinzato eating that explained her 104 years of bounding exuberance? While she may not have seen this as a pertinent question, researchers have been seeking answers to it. Craig and Bradley Willcox's work includes meticulous data collection and offers important insights. They began by noting the time span within which today's Okinawan centenarians have lived. All Okinawans age 100 or more who are alive today were born between 1903 and 1914. During the first third of their lives, roughly before 1940, the vast majority of the calories they consumed—more than 60 percent—came from one food: the *imo,* or Okinawan sweet potato.

A purple or yellow variety related to our orange sweet potato, the imo came here from the Americas about 400 years ago and took well to Okinawan soils. That was lucky for pre–World War II Okinawans, who were otherwise calorie starved. This sweet potato—high in flavonoids, vitamin C, fiber, carotenoids, and slow-burning carbohydrates—is one of the healthiest foods on the planet.

In fact, the traditional Okinawan diet was about 80 percent carbohydrates, the Willcoxes found. Before 1940 Okinawans also consumed fish at least three times per week together with seven servings of vegetables and maybe one or two servings of grain per day. They also ate two servings of flavonoid-rich soy, usually in the form of tofu. They didn't eat much fruit; they enjoyed a few eggs a week.

Dairy and meat represented only about 3 percent of their calories. Never influenced by Buddhism, 20th-century Okinawans observed no taboos against eating meat, but they still only ate it rarely. On special occasions, usually during the Lunar New Year, people butchered the family pig and feasted on pork—probably an important protein source at the time. A typical traditional meal of the time, wrote the Willcoxes in an article they authored for the *Journal of the American College of Nutrition*, began with Okinawan-style miso soup including seaweed, tofu, sweet potato, and green leafy vegetables. The main dish was *champuru,* stir-fried vegetables that might include goya, daikon (radish), Chinese okra, pumpkin, burdock root, or green papaya, sometimes accompanied by smaller servings of fish, meat, or noodles prepared with herbs, spices, and cooking oil. To drink, they served freshly brewed *sanpin* (jasmine) tea and perhaps a little locally brewed *awamori* (millet brandy).

Three foods in the Okinawan diet of those days—turmeric, sweet potato, and seaweed—provided an additional benefit we understand better today: They mimic *caloric restriction,* a digestive survival mode that has longevity benefits. As food is digested, mitochondria in our cells convert calories into energy. A by-product of this process are free radicals, oxidizing agents that deteriorate the body from the inside out just as oxidation forms rust on iron and ultimately destroys it. Free radicals can stiffen the arteries, shrink the brain, and wrinkle the skin. In caloric restriction mode, our cells protect themselves by producing less energy but also throwing off fewer free radicals and thus slowing the aging process. One way to turn on caloric restriction is to eat about 40 percent fewer calories than the average American consumes (about 2,500 for a man and 1,800 for a woman.) But recent research from the Willcoxes has shown that regular consumption of turmeric, sweet potato, and seaweed can provide some of the benefits of caloric restriction, tripping genetic triggers that minimize production of free radicals without causing hunger.

Typical Daily Diet of Okinawans, 1949
(Percentage of daily intake in grams)

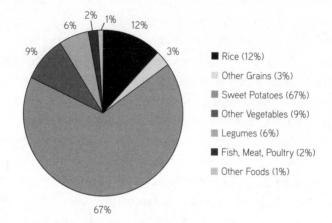

- ■ Rice (12%)
- ■ Other Grains (3%)
- ■ Sweet Potatoes (67%)
- ■ Other Vegetables (9%)
- ■ Legumes (6%)
- ■ Fish, Meat, Poultry (2%)
- ■ Other Foods (1%)

Source: Willcox et al. [1].

Typical Daily Diet of Okinawans, 1989
(Percentage of daily intake in grams)

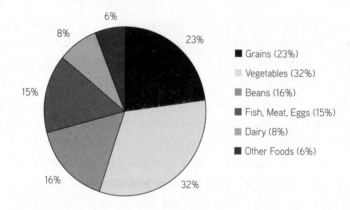

- ■ Grains (23%)
- ■ Vegetables (32%)
- ■ Beans (16%)
- ■ Fish, Meat, Eggs (15%)
- ■ Dairy (8%)
- ■ Other Foods (6%)

Source: Adapted from Akisaka et al.

Through the post-war decades, Okinawans ate more greens and more yellow, orange, and red vegetables than other Japanese. They also ate more meat—primarily pork—but they ate less fish, less salt, and much less added sugar.

FAST-FOOD INVASION

As healthful as they were, some of these Okinawan food traditions foundered mid-century. Following the war, the United States established an army base in the middle of Okinawa. Western influences—and economic prosperity—crept into traditional life and food habits changed. According to detailed Japanese government surveys, sweet potatoes dropped from 60 percent to fewer than 5 percent of Okinawans' daily calories between 1949 and 1960. Meanwhile, they doubled their rice consumption, and bread, virtually unknown before, also crept in. Milk consumption increased; meat, eggs, and poultry consumption increased more than sevenfold. Not coincidentally, cancers of the lung, breast, and colon almost doubled.

The meat in their diet gave me pause. When I first struck off on my Blue Zones research in 2000, I was absolutely convinced that I'd find that a vegan diet yielded the greatest health and life expectancy. So when I discovered that older Okinawans not only ate pork but loved it, I thought their example must be an outlier—that they were living long *despite* pork. Pork is high in saturated fat, which, when consumed in excess, often leads to heart disease. But again, we learn a few lessons. Okinawans stewed the pork for days, cooking out and skimming off the fat. What they ate, in the end, was the high-protein collagen.

One dietary expert I met in Okinawa, Kazuhilo Taira, believed that it was this pork protein that actually explained their longevity. His theory was that we all suffer small tears in the blood vessels that bring blood to our brains. Severe tears result in strokes, but minor tears, while still doing damage, often go unnoticed. Pork protein actually acted like a caulking of sorts, for the pig protein is very similar to human protein. And it was this protein that Okinawans love.

"Oh yes, I like meat, but not always," Shinzato had told me. "When I was a girl, I ate it only during New Year festivals. I'm not in the habit of eating it every day."

But today fast-food restaurants serving quick-cooked burgers and other meat sandwiches abound in Okinawa. The island boasts the largest A&W Root Beer stand in the world. In 2005 Okinawans, who live on an island only 70 miles long and 7 miles wide, consumed tons of Spam, a processed meat product introduced by American GIs after World War II. Between 1949 and 1972 Okinawans' daily intake increased by 400 calories. They were consuming more than 200 calories per day *more* than they needed—like Americans. And health statistics show the effect of those changes. By 2000 Okinawa ranked 26th among Japan's 47 prefectures for life expectancy of men at birth, while older Okinawans, whose diets had solidified before that time period, are the world's longest-lived people.

Some traditions do not die—and apparently some food traditions keep Okinawans living long and healthy lives, even with the onslaught of the modern fast-food culture.

TOP LONGEVITY FOODS FROM OKINAWA

Okinawans have long told their children to eat something from the land and from the sea every day. I've found that these time-honored adages survive for a reason, as do other food traditions that help contribute to a long, healthy life.

BITTER MELONS The bitter melon is not a fruit as its name implies—it's a long, knobby gourd that looks something like a warty cucumber. Eaten green, it tastes quite bitter. Known as goya in Okinawa, bitter melon is often served with other vegetables in a stir-fried dish called *goya champuru,* the national dish and cornerstone of the Okinawan diet. Recent studies found bitter melon an "effective anti-diabetic" as powerful as pharmaceuticals in helping to regulate blood sugar. Like the sweet potato, turmeric, and seaweed common to the Okinawan diet, goya contains chemicals that may slow the production of corrosive free radicals. Bitter melon is more and more often available in American gourmet produce markets. There is nothing quite like it as a substitute in our everyday cuisine.

TOFU Tofu is to Okinawans what bread is to the French and potatoes are to Eastern Europeans: a daily habit. Okinawans eat about eight times more tofu than Americans do today. Made by curdling soy milk to coagulate the bean's protein, the product is then pressed into a block and sliced like a piece of cake. Along with other soy products, tofu is renowned for helping to protect the heart. Studies show that people who eat soy products in place of meat have lower cholesterol and triglyceride levels, which reduce their risk of heart disease.

SWEET POTATOES Okinawan imo is a supercharged purple sweet potato, a cousin of the yellow-orange sweet varieties. Despite its sweet, satisfying taste, the supercharged purple imo does not spike blood sugar as much as a regular white potato. The leaves are eaten as greens in miso soup; the potato itself has been a staple since the 17th century. Like other sweet potatoes, it contains antioxidants called sporamin, which possess a variety of potent antiaging properties. But the purple version is higher in antioxidants than its cousins.

GARLIC Sometimes eaten pickled on Okinawa, garlic is one of nature's most powerful natural medicines. A recent review of thousands of scientific studies concluded that "intake of garlic by humans may either prevent or decrease the incidence of major chronic diseases associated with old age" and named atherosclerosis, stroke, cancer, immune disorders, cerebral aging, arthritis, and cataract formation among those diseases.

TURMERIC Ginger's golden cousin, turmeric, figures prominently in the Okinawan diet as both a spice and a tea. A powerful anticancer, antioxidant, and anti-inflammatory agent, turmeric contains several compounds now under study for their antiaging properties, especially the ability to mimic caloric restriction in the body. Its compound curcumin has been shown in both clinical and population studies to slow the progression of dementia—which may explain why Okinawans suffer lower rates of Alzheimer's disease than Americans do. The Okinawan practice of adding black pepper to turmeric increases the bioavailability of curcumin 1,000 times.

BROWN RICE In Okinawa, where centenarians eat rice *every* day, both brown and white rice are enjoyed. Nutritionally, brown rice is superior. The milling done to produce white rice strips away dietary fiber and nutrients, including most of the B vitamins and all of the essential fatty acids found in rice. Okinawan brown rice, tastier than the brown rice we know, is soaked in water to germinate until it just begins to sprout, unlocking enzymes that break down sugar and protein and giving the rice a sweet flavor and softer texture.

GREEN TEA Okinawans drink a special kind of green tea they call *shan-pien,* which translates to "tea with a bit of a scent," created by adding jasmine flowers and often a little turmeric. Green tea contains unique substances that studies suggest may protect against a host of age-related problems, including various forms of heart disease and cancer, stroke, osteoporosis, diabetes, and mental decline.

SHIITAKE MUSHROOMS These smoky-flavored fungi, which grow naturally on dead bark in forests, help flavor Okinawans's customary miso soup and stir-fries. They contain more than 100 different compounds with immune-protecting properties. Purchased dried, they can be reconstituted by soaking or by cooking in a liquid like a soup or sauce, and most of their nutritional value remains.

SEAWEEDS (KOMBU AND WAKAME) Seaweeds in general provide a filling, low-calorie, nutrient-rich boost to the diet. Kombu and wakame are the most common seaweeds eaten in Okinawa, enhancing many soups and stews. Rich in carotenoids, folate, magnesium, iron, calcium, and iodine, they also possess at least six compounds found only in sea plants that seem to serve as effective antioxidants at the cellular level. Wakame, an edible seaweed harvested for centuries in Japan and Korea, is now available dried in the United States. Kombu, a type of kelp, is also a centuries-old Asian mainstay now sold dried and packaged in the United States.

For recipes from Okinawa, see pages 255–265.

CHAPTER THREE

࿓

A Diet From the World's Longest-Lived Men: Sardinia, Italy

F OR MOST OF THE PAST CENTURY members of the Melis family have started each day with an egg fried in lard, a piece of sourdough bread to soak up the yolk, a glass of goat's milk, and two cups of coffee. Then the men strike off over the rocky, thistle-clumped terrain surrounding their village, Perdasdefogu, to pasture their sheep, while the women stay behind to mind the children, tend the garden, wash clothes in the river, mill grain, and bake bread.

At noon, lunch centers on a bowl of savory bean-and-vegetable minestrone soup garnished with a dollop of lard and a piece of bread washed down with a glass of deep-red Cannonau wine. An early dinner begins with leftover soup, segueing to seasonal garden vegetables, more bread, hard pecorino cheese, and, occasionally, a small piece of larded pork— again accompanied by the wine. While pork, white bread, eggs, and lard might not sound like the hallmarks of a longevity diet, it has worked for the nine brothers and sisters of the Melis family. They hold the Guinness world record for the highest combined age of any nine siblings: a total of 828 years. In August 2013, the eldest sister, Consolata, turned 106.

The Melis family lives on the Italian island of Sardinia, in the middle of the Mediterranean, almost equidistant from France, Italy, and North

Africa. Here 42,000 people, descendants of a Bronze Age culture, occupy the rocky slopes of the Supramonte mountains in villages that festoon the hills like a giant string of pearls. Several thousand years ago their forebears were pushed into the rugged hills by Phoenician and Roman invaders. Unlike the landscape of coastal Sardinia, much of which is fertile farmland, these inland slopes are menacingly steep, sun-beaten, and blanketed with prickly vegetation. Nevertheless, the villages of the Ogliastra region produce more male centenarians, proportionally speaking, than anywhere else on Earth. In one village, Villagrande, not far from the Melis' home, 5 centenarians still live among 2,500 people. In America, only 1 in about 5,000 people reaches age 100.

Not long ago I spent several weeks wandering the 14 whitewashed villages of this Blue Zone, trying to tease out details about their longevity diet. I spent three days wandering the hills with a 28-year-old shepherd who had learned his skills from his great-grandfather. Because pasturing animals over this sparse terrain required days of provisions, he had learned to travel light with foods that wouldn't spoil. His diet: unleavened *carta di musica* bread, dried fava beans, pecorino cheese made from his own sheep's milk, and a generous supply of the local Cannonau wine.

Near the village of Silanus I met Tonino Tola, a robust 75-year-old shepherd with arms like oak limbs, a vise-grip handshake, and a gladiator's profile. I shadowed him for a day, watching him butcher animals with an ax and herd goats in the hills, sometimes tucking a straggler under each arm. At day's end he invited me into his house for a snack. We ducked into his low-ceilinged kitchen. His wife, Giovanna, a heavy-set woman with quick, intelligent eyes, offered me wine or coffee and set out *papassini*—a feast day cookie made from raisins, grape juice, almonds, and fennel. "So this is what men here eat to grow so big and strong?" I asked. Tonino laughed.

I assumed that, given Sardinia's pastoral roots and the close interdependence of people and animals, meat was a cornerstone of their diet. But Tonino corrected me. Most days, he said, he drank sheep's milk and ate Sicilian bread, fava beans, lard, and "what my garden produced." In the summer he and his family mostly ate zucchini, tomatoes, potatoes, eggplants, and, most significantly, fava beans. Meat was, at best, a weekly affair, boiled on Sunday with pasta or roasted during festivals. Families typically sold their animals to buy grain staples. In the winter they almost never ate meat. The sheep only ate grass and herbs. "They were very skinny," Tonino said. "It wasn't worth it to kill them."

In most parts of the world, for every one guy who makes it to 100, there are five women who do too. (Good news, single men: Your dating odds improve as you get older.) But in this region of Sardinia, the ratio is one to one. And it's not because women die young here, but rather because men elude heart disease longer—and probably better than men anywhere else in the world. For most of the past 2,000 years villagers here have lived in relative isolation from the rest of the island. (The first paved roads to the region were carved through in the 1960s.) Because the cropland is so difficult, people have had to scrape together a living by tending sheep and growing small gardens. Meanwhile, women care for children, repair the leaky roof, and handle all the finances and business negotiations. In the past women were even in charge of defense, leading the armed response to lowland intruders. They bear much of the day-to-day stress, which may help explain why men here live so long.

When you ask Sardinian centenarians to explain why they have lived so long, they'll frequently tell you it's the clean air, the locally produced wine, or, as one centenarian suggested, because they "make love every Sunday." Elders here are considered cultural treasures who accrue esteem with age by holding the living memory of the culture. Older people don't retire on Sardinia as much as they shift jobs. Men may stop tending their sheep, but they'll put their efforts and talents to work in the villages. It's not uncommon to see 90-year-olds working as walking patrols or advising city government. In turn, the expectation that they should contribute something to society gets them out of bed in the morning and keeps them out of the easy chair, staying active and using their brains. By and large they don't retreat to retirement homes or senior communities. When I asked the daughter of a mentally frail 103-year-old man if she considered putting him in an old-age home, she glared at me and said, "That would shame our family."

To find out what Sardinians actually did to become centenarians, our team's Sardinian collaborator, Gianni Pes, examined lifestyle surveys conducted with more than 200 centenarians throughout the island. He learned that pastoralism, as he called it, was most highly correlated with reaching age 100. Shepherds who wandered the island's highlands, moving livestock from the mountains to the plains, were up to ten times more likely to live to 100 than men in the rest of Italy, including farmers, whose lives also involved seasons of exhausting labor. Pes postulated that farmers may overwork in the growing season, leading to higher rates of inflammation. (Working too hard triggers inflammation, much the way an injury does.) We might think of shepherds as having the easier job compared to the peasants, who were thought to work much harder. But now it seems that a shepherd's regular, low-intensity physical effort—slowly walking up and down the mountain slopes—might provide a better model for the type of exercise that the rest of us should be doing.

The second most highly associated factor for reaching age 100, Pes discovered, was the hilliness of the terrain—and how far one walked to work. The steeper the terrain, the longer you tended to live. The shepherds on Sardinia were gently walking up and down hills all day long—not just in the pastures but also in their villages. Every trip to the store, to church, or to the local bar occasioned a mildly strenuous climb.

THE SARDINIAN DIET

Searching the archives for food surveys carried out in Sardinia during the 20th century, Pes found nutritional data published in the early 1930s by Italian hygienist C. Fermi, information reflecting the lifestyle of Sardinia's population long before dietary habits changed in the 1960s with the arrival of paved roads and generally improved economic conditions, sanitation, and public health. According to Fermi, all variables were collected through a structured questionnaire completed by public health personnel in each village. He found that in a month, people living in the Sardinian hills consumed only 3 servings of meat and 1 ounce of nuts, but also 11 pounds of wheat, 16 pounds of barley, 1 pound of cheese, and 7 liters of wine.

In 1938 another dietary researcher, G. Peretti, visited 28 farming families and 17 shepherd families living in three Sardinian villages. Overall, he found that more than 65 percent of the calories residents consumed came from carbohydrates such as bread, pastas, potatoes, or beans. Fat accounted for about 20 percent of their diet, mostly from animal sources such as goat's milk or sheep's cheese but also from olive oil. The other 15 percent of the diet was protein, three-quarters from plants, mostly beans. Americans tend to think that more protein is good for us. But here was a long-lived population that grew up on a low-protein diet. Recent research points to potential benefits from such a diet: A study at the Davis School of Gerontology showed that a low-protein diet is associated with lower rates of diabetes, cancer, and death for people under 65. Incredibly, for people between 50 and 65, those in the higher protein category had a 73-fold increase in diabetes risk and were more than four times as likely to die of cancer. For people over 65, the findings flipped: Those with high protein intake had a 28 percent reduction in mortality.

Potatoes were the next most important vegetable in the Sardinian diet, followed by tomatoes, onions, zucchini, and cabbage. Peretti noted only two fruits: pears and cherries. Sardinians ate about 15 pounds of cheese and 50 pounds of barley per year, he recorded. The meat they ate came mainly from sheep or occasionally pigs and chickens (mostly reserved for holidays), but never from fish. Sardinia is an island, but for residents of the highlands, the sea was a two-day round-trip journey rarely made. Wine contributed about 110 calories, or about two small glasses, to the diet of Sardinians each day. In sum, Sardinians consumed 2,720 calories per day—about what an American consumes today—but their physical activity warranted this high caloric intake.

Over the years, the Sardinian diet evolved. As roads and electricity came in during the 1960s, so did Italian influences like a taste for pasta and sweets, and a wider variety of fruits—along with the prosperity to afford them. Frozen vegetables and noodles started appearing in daily minestrone. Olive oil, while always consumed in this Blue Zone, increasingly

Typical Daily Diet of Sardinian Shepherds, 1943
(Percentage of daily intake in grams)

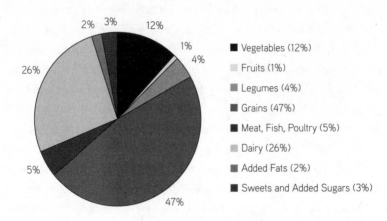

Source: Adapted from Peretti, 1943, as presented in Carbini [1].

Meat and dairy are almost entirely from sheep and goats. Average daily wine consumption of 114 grams (4 ounces) is not included.

replaced lard as the main fat used for cooking. Meat, always associated with wealth, also increased in popularity. No coincidence, then, that obesity rates, diabetes, and heart disease have also soared in recent decades. Pes found that after 1950 Sardinians began to eat more. They replaced beans and potato consumption dropped about 40 percent, while consumption of higher-calorie foods like beef and fish increased by about 50 percent. Counterintuitively, perhaps, lard consumption dropped by 80 percent.

TOP LONGEVITY FOODS FROM SARDINIA

Many of the same Mediterranean foods that explain longevity in Ikaria also explain longevity in Sardinia. Olive oil, lemons, beans, and greens are common to both, and the Sardinian diet includes a few other longevity foods we can all benefit from eating.

GOAT'S MILK AND SHEEP'S MILK Both have higher nutritional value and are more easily digested than cow's milk. A recent study in the *European Journal of Clinical Nutrition* showed that both sheep's milk and goat's milk lower bad cholesterol, are anti-inflammatory, and may protect against cardiovascular disease and colon cancer. The higher calcium and phosphorus content of goat's milk may have helped people living in the Sardinian Blue Zones preserve their bone density and consequently lower their risk of fractures. Goat's milk is also rich in zinc and selenium, which are essential for optimal immune system activity and to promote healthy aging. The sharp pecorino cheese made from fermented sheep's milk in Sardinia is particularly interesting. Because of its rich flavor, it can be used sparingly in pastas, soups, and grated over vegetables. Since pecorino is made from the milk of grass-fed sheep, it has high levels of omega-3 fatty acids.

FLAT BREAD *(carta di musica)* The most common bread consumed by Sardinian shepherds is a dry, flat bread made of high-protein, low-gluten *Triticum* durum wheat (the main ingredient in Italian pasta). High in fiber and complex carbohydrates, it does not cause a sugar spike in blood like processed or refined grains do and it's easier on the pancreas, lowering the risk for type 2 diabetes. Its name comes from the observation that it is flat and thin, like music paper. Another traditional flat bread is *pane carasau*. This thin, flat bread made of durum wheat flour, salt, yeast, and water was invented for shepherds, who pastured their sheep for months at a time. It can last up to a year. Whole durum wheat has a low to medium glycemic score, and so it doesn't spike blood sugar. It also contains only a fraction of the gluten that white bread does.

BARLEY Ground into flour or added to soups, barley was found to be the food most highly associated with living to 100 among Sardinian men. Barley bread *(orgiathu)* was favored by shepherds because of its long shelf life and looked much like a regular loaf of bread but was made of ground barley. This bread has a much lower glycemic index than wheat bread, meaning it increases blood glucose more slowly than wheat bread does and thus puts less stress on the pancreas and kidneys. We don't know if it does that because of barley's high protein, magnesium, and fiber content (much higher than oatmeal) or because it was pushing other less healthy foods (such as white wheat flour) out of the diet. Ironically, barley was considered a poor man's food until recently, when it has made a comeback in Sardinian haute cuisine.

SOURDOUGH BREAD *(moddizzosu)* Much like sourdough bread in the United States, Sardinian sourdough breads are made from whole wheat and use live lactobacilli (rather than yeast) to rise the dough. This process also converts sugars and gluten into lactic acid, lowering the bread's glycemic index and imparting a pleasant, faintly sour taste. Pes has demonstrated that this type of bread is able to lower the glycemic load, reducing after-meal glucose and insulin blood levels by 25 percent. This helps protect the pancreas and may help prevent obesity and diabetes.

FENNEL Fennel's licorice taste flavors several Sardinian dishes. It's used as a vegetable (the bulb), as an herb (its willowy fronds), and as a spice (its seeds) and is rich in fiber and soluble vitamins such as A, B, and C. It's also a good diuretic; therefore, it helps to maintain the blood pressure low.

FAVA BEANS AND CHICKPEAS Eaten in soups and stews, fava beans and chickpeas play an important part in the Sardinian diet, delivering protein and fiber. They are one of the foods most highly associated with reaching age 100.

TOMATOES Sardinian tomato sauce (for recipe, see page 270) tops breads and pizzas and is the base for several pasta dishes. Tomatoes are a rich source of vitamin C and potassium. Cooking tomatoes breaks down their cell walls, making lycopene and other antioxidants more available. The Sardinian custom of coupling olive oil with tomatoes (either drizzling it over raw tomatoes or using it to make sauces) further increases the body's ability to absorb nutrients and antioxidants.

ALMONDS Almonds, associated with Mediterranean cooking everywhere, appear regularly in Sardinian cooking, eaten alone, chopped into main dishes, or ground into a paste for desserts. One study showed that almonds included in a low-calorie diet helped people lose more weight and belly fat while they experienced an increase in protective high-density lipoprotein (HDL) cholesterol and a drop in systolic blood pressure (the top number).

MILK THISTLE Sardinians drink a tea of milk thistle, a native wild plant, to, as locals believe, "cleanse the liver." Emerging research suggests that the milk thistle's main active ingredient, silymarin, is an antioxidant and has anti-inflammatory benefits. It can be found in American health food stories as an ingredient in some herbal teas and in capsule and tablet form.

CANNONAU WINE Sardinia's distinctive garnet red Cannonau wine is made from the sun-stressed Grenache grape. When I first traveled there, I was hoping to discover a longevity elixir in this wine. Sardinians drink three to four small (three-ounce) glasses of wine a day on average, spread out between breakfast, lunch, dinner, and a late afternoon social hour in the village. One might argue that the all-day small doses of this antioxidant-rich beverage could explain fewer heart attacks. Dry red wines in general offer the same health advantage.

For recipes from Sardinia, see pages 265–279.

CHAPTER FOUR

❧

An American
Blue Zones Diet:
Loma Linda, California

A T MIDMORNING ON ANY GIVEN DAY, Ellsworth Wareham presides over a breakfast of biblical proportions. Spread out on the kitchen table before him at his home in Loma Linda, California, is a giant bowl of whole-grain cereal floating in soy milk, a cornucopia-like fruit bowl, a stack of whole-grain toast with nut butter, a large glass of full-pulp orange juice, and a handful of nuts. From his kitchen window he commands a view of orange groves and the waves of smoky brown foothills that ascend to the snowcapped San Jacinto Mountains.

Later in the day, around 4 p.m., Wareham will resume his place at the kitchen table. This time it will be to tuck into his second—and only other—meal of the day: mounds of beans, raw vegetables, cooked asparagus, cabbage, and broccoli, finished with a handful of nuts and dates for dessert—the exact diet, he might add, that God prescribed for the garden of Eden. And, as one of America's largest and most robust epidemiology studies has shown, it's also the healthiest diet for humankind today.

I first met Wareham in 2005, when I was researching an article about longevity for *National Geographic* magazine. I'd sought him out because he seemed to be an iconic Seventh-day Adventist, following a branch of Christianity whose members live longer than any other Americans. Seventh-day

Adventists are conservative Protestants who distinguish themselves from other Christians in that they evangelize with health and celebrate the Sabbath on Saturday instead of Sunday. From sunset on Friday until sunset on Saturday, every week, Seventh-day Adventists create a "sanctuary in time," spending most of the 24 hours in quiet contemplation or attending church and avoiding TV, movies, and other distractions. At midday on Saturday after church they join other Adventists for potluck lunches. Later in the afternoon, they strike out with friends and family on a nature walk for healthy doses of sunshine and fresh air. They shun smoking, drinking, and dancing.

It was a hot September afternoon, but Wareham was outside, hard at work, when I first walked into his yard to introduce myself. He'd been building a fence along a hillside, struggling to corkscrew a pole digger through the rocky soil. When he saw me he stood up, wiped his brow with his forearm, squeegeeing sweat down onto his clinging T-shirt and muscled pectorals. "Well, it's a pleasure to meet you, Dan," he said genteelly, extending a strong hand. He had erected two posts, each of which required digging a two-foot hole, pouring cement, and squaring off a forty-pound pole. Judging by the imposing pile of poles in the middle of the yard, he still had work to do. "It'll get done in a few days," he told me confidently.

Four days later Wareham was at his post in the operating room, assisting the lead cardiac surgeon. An early pioneer in open-heart surgery, he'd been working on people's hearts for 47 years, performing three to four surgeries per week, some lasting up to six hours. In the late 1950s he'd started the cardiac surgery program at Loma Linda University and retired from there in 1985. Lately, he'd been making the four-hour round-trip each day in his compact Toyota to one of the two hospitals where he now assists. In fact, the epiphany that had led him to adopt the Adventist lifestyle had come to him when he was at work in an operating room.

"In the early days we'd need to connect the arterial line into the leg artery. Later it would be straight into the aorta," he said. In his work clothes he'd looked like an affable grandpa, but now in scrubs he looked decidedly professorial. Tall and lean, he wore wide-rimmed glasses and had a mustache. "I observed when I was cutting down into the legs of these patients that those who were vegetarians had better arteries—smooth and supple." Nonvegetarians, he said, tended to have a lot of heavy calcium and plaques in their arteries. "I began thinking about it. And I saw people getting their toes cut off or their feet cut off because of vascular disease, and that motivated me. At middle age, I decided to become a vegan. With the exception of an occasional piece of fish, all I eat are plants."

GOD'S FOOD GUIDELINES

In support of a biblical diet of grains, fruits, nuts, and vegetables, Adventists cite Genesis 1:29: "And God said, Behold, I have given you every herb bearing seed, which is upon the face of all the earth, and every tree, in the which is the fruit of a tree yielding seed; to you it shall be for meat." The Adventists encourage a "well-balanced diet" including nuts, fruits, and legumes, low in sugar, salt, and refined grains. Their diet prohibits foods deemed "unclean" by the Bible, such as pork or shellfish. The only beverage endorsed is water, at least six glasses a day.

Today the Adventist diet in its current interpretation is demonstrably yielding the healthiest Americans. It is a plant-based diet that emphasizes nuts, whole grains, beans, and soy products. It's also very low in sugar, salt, and refined grain. It includes small amounts of meat, dairy, and eggs, and discourages coffee and alcohol. A new study has found that adherents have the nation's lowest rates of heart disease and diabetes and very low rates of obesity. They also live up to a decade longer than the rest of us.

Gary Fraser, of Loma Linda University, probably understands the Adventists' lifestyle better than anybody else alive. Trained as a cardiologist and epidemiologist, and an Adventist himself, he has for the past 12 years directed the Adventist Health Studies, an enormous project entailing several studies that has tracked tens of thousands of Adventists for decades. In simple terms, the study asks scores of questions about what people eat, and then follows them long enough until they develop heart disease, cancer, or die. Looking back on the data, Fraser can see which diets are associated with shorter or longer life spans. He can also cite the cause of death, whether it's heart disease, cancer, diabetes, or stroke.

The first Adventist Health Study, the AHS-1, funded by the National Institutes of Health, followed 34,000 Adventists in California for 14 years. In that study, Fraser calculated that Adventists who most strictly followed the religion's teachings lived about ten years longer than people who didn't. The practices most likely to yield that longevity? Fraser winnowed them down to five, each adding about two years to life expectancy:

- Eating a plant-based diet with only small amounts of dairy or fish
- Not smoking
- Maintaining medium body weight
- Eating a handful of nuts four to five times per week
- Doing regular physical activity

Think about this for a moment. These are Americans. They live among us, drive by the same fast-food restaurants, shop in the same grocery stores, breathe the same air, and work in the same jobs we do. But they're living up to a decade longer than the rest of us!

In 2002 Fraser and his colleagues launched a second, even more ambitious study. The Adventist Health Study 2 (AHS-2) recruited 96,000 men and women of all ethnicities. It asked each participant at least 500 questions about their health histories, eating habits, and physical activity, among other topics. To figure out how diet impacted how long people lived, Frazer and his colleagues broke the study subjects into four general categories: (1) vegans, (2) ovo-lacto vegetarians (vegetarians who consume eggs and dairy, (3) pesco-vegetarians (vegetarians who eat fish and very little meat), and (4) nonvegetarians.

They gleaned several insights. Meat-eaters, for one thing, tended to consume more soda pop, desserts, and refined grains than vegetarians. They also tended to be fatter. If you were to take two men of equal height, one a meat-eater and the other a vegan, the meat-eater was likely to weigh an extra 20 pounds. The meat-eater was also likely to die sooner.

Although vegans tended to weigh less, they didn't live the longest, the study found. That distinction went to pesco-vegetarians, or pescatarians, those who ate a plant-based diet with up to one serving of fish per day.

TYPICAL DAILY DIET OF
SEVENTH-DAY ADVENTISTS

When a prominent medical journal published the results of Fraser's study, I phoned Wareham. I was interested in his take on the article, but mostly I wondered how he, as a practitioner of the Adventist diet, had managed to stick with it for more than half a century. Most diets fail after nine months.

"All human tastes, except mother's milk, are acquired," he told me from his kitchen phone. He was now 99 years old and, although he had given up surgery, he was still in perfect health. "You start by eating a little bit of plant-based food and grow with it. You keep eating it and pretty soon you start to enjoy it."

Typical Daily Diet of Seventh-Day Adventists
(Percentage of daily intake in grams)

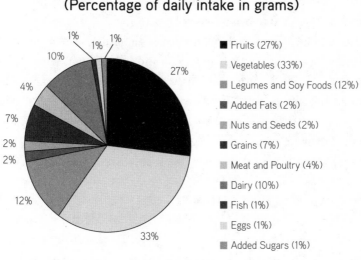

- Fruits (27%)
- Vegetables (33%)
- Legumes and Soy Foods (12%)
- Added Fats (2%)
- Nuts and Seeds (2%)
- Grains (7%)
- Meat and Poultry (4%)
- Dairy (10%)
- Fish (1%)
- Eggs (1%)
- Added Sugars (1%)

Source: Jaceldo-Siegl et al. [1].

This chart represents the average intake of various food groups for the Adventists participating in Adventist Health Study 2. The data tables included 513 in the white cohort and 414 in the black cohort. The averages used for this table were weighted proportionally in combining the data to reflect a more accurate average for the total population.

He told me that eating only two meals a day helps him to keep his weight down. "I love to eat," he said. "When I eat, I eat a lot, and I really enjoy it. So twice daily is enough." He almost never eats out at restaurants unless he gets a hankering for salmon. Nuts are usually part of the menu. "I know walnuts are supposed to be good, but I also enjoy peanuts and cashews and almonds. Purists will tell you to eat them raw but salted is okay too—whatever is handy," he said. " And you know I'm very much against sugar except natural sources like fruit, dates, or figs. I never eat refined sugar or drink sodas."

Wareham prefers to drink water, a beverage he claims keeps the weight off. He drinks at least two glasses when he first gets up. "I want to make sure before I get busy and forget," he said. Then he keeps drinking water throughout the day. "One of my little rituals is to never pass a water fountain without having a little drink."

As Wareham described his diet, I was thinking that it sounded pretty bland, the type of food that might excite a rabbit, and I told him so. "Once you get used to being a vegetarian, the very idea of eating a cow's secretion or an animal's muscle is much less appealing," he replied.

I asked him if he ever thought about mortality, about dying. "Well, Dan, I do," he said. "When we first met, I remember you asking me if I would ever get to age 100 and now I'm pretty sure I will. I feel good. My mind is sharp. I still mow the lawn. If I have any problems, I'm not aware of them."

I told him I was writing a new book and asked him how I should describe how he feels to readers.

"Tell them I still feel like I'm 20," he said

TOP ADVENTIST LONGEVITY FOODS

AVOCADOS High in potassium and low in salt, avocados may help reduce blood pressure and the risk of stroke. Ounce for ounce, an avocado contains 30 percent more potassium than a banana, a dietary staple for many people with high blood pressure.

SALMON The longest-lived Adventists are pesco-vegetarians. They eat plant-based food and up to one serving of fish per day, most often salmon, well known for its heart-healthy properties. Researchers at the Harvard School of Public Health recently concluded that people who eat one to two three-ounce servings weekly of fish rich in omega-3 fatty acids—the oil that collects in the fatty tissue of cold-water fish—reduced their chance of dying from a heart attack by a third. To play it on the safest side, look for wild-caught Alaska salmon, which contains the least contaminants and the most omega-3 fatty acid–rich oils.

NUTS A study during the 1990s found that Adventists who ate a handful of nuts at least five times a week lived two to three years longer than people who didn't eat any nuts. More research since then found links between nut-eaters and lower rates of cholesterol, blood pressure, chronic inflammation, diabetes, and myriad other troubles that add up to cardiovascular disease.

BEANS For vegetarian Adventists, beans and other legumes such as lentils and peas represent important daily protein sources. There are at least 70 varieties of beans to choose from and an infinite number of ways to prepare them.

WATER Ellen G. White, founder of the Adventist Church, prescribed six to eight glasses of water daily. Apart from its well-known hydrating and toxin-flushing benefits, water consumption promotes better blood flow and less chance of clotting, some studies have suggested. Beyond their health value, six glasses of water a day likely pushes diet sodas, fruit juices, and other sugar-sweetened or artificially sweetened beverages out of the diet.

OATMEAL A staple for Adventists, slow-cooked oatmeal is frequently mentioned as the breakfast for American centenarians everywhere. It provides a balanced portion of fats, complex carbohydrates, and plant protein, along with good doses of iron and B vitamins. Its high fiber content makes it filling, and nuts and dried fruits can add fiber, flavor, and variety.

WHOLE WHEAT BREAD Like other Americans, Adventists often find themselves eating lunch at school, at work, or on the go. Slices of 100 percent whole wheat bread are convenient and healthy "packaging" for protein and vegetable fillings, such as avocado or nut butters. True 100 percent whole wheat breads add only 70 calories per slice to the sandwich plus small amounts of a wide variety of nutrients. The high fiber content minimizes the need for mid-afternoon snacking, which is often less than healthy.

SOY MILK Adventists use real soy milk (not the sweetened, flavored variety) as a topping for breakfast cereals, a whitener for herbal teas, and an all-around healthy alternative to dairy. High in protein and low in fat, soy milk contains phytoestrogens that may protect against certain types of cancer. Because it's so versatile, it can figure into daily breakfast, lunch, and dinner.

For Adventist recipes, see pages 279–287.

CHAPTER FIVE

☙

History's Best Longevity Diet: Nicoya Peninsula, Costa Rica

W HEN I FIRST MET FRANCESCA "PANCHITA" CASTILLO, she was standing in her front yard, wearing a frilly pink carnival dress and swinging a four-foot-long machete. With vigorous, violent blows, the 99-year-old beat back the branches and low-lying bush of the encroaching jungle—the equivalent of my mowing the lawn back in Minneapolis. When she caught sight of me, she stopped, stood up straight, and serenely watched me climb the dirt path leading to her wooden shack. She didn't know me, or my business, yet when I reached her, she took my hand in both of hers, looked up at me with her cocoa brown, sweat-glistened face, and unleashed a whoop of joy.

"How can I serve you?" she said by way of greeting.

Since then, during two Blue Zones expeditions to Nicoya, Costa Rica, I have often visited Castillo, now 107, in part to learn how she'd maintained machete-wielding vitality for more than a century, but mostly because I just liked her. The carnival dress, I discovered, was both a daily uniform and a manifestation of an irrepressibly joyful spirit.

One day, when my colleague Elizabeth Lopez, a psychologist based in Costa Rica, and I were interviewing her about her diet, Castillo grew tired of our questions, grabbed my arm, and said, "Come." We followed her into her kitchen, a low, dirt-floored room flanked by wooden counters built around an enormous *fogón,* a wood-burning stove made of clay used by the region's indigenous Chorotega Indians. I looked around. A bowl of bananas and papayas sat on the counter for easy access. Below, out of sight behind a cloth, Castillo stored beans, onions, garlic, and cooking oil. She kept only fresh cheese and tomatoes in her refrigerator. She had no packaged or processed foods; everything required preparation except the cheese and fresh fruit.

Castillo got busy. Working with slow, deliberate movements and oblivious to us watching her, she stoked the oven, blew on some coals still hot from breakfast, and produced a bright flame. Then she covered the fire with a sheet of pounded steel that would serve as a griddle of sorts. Earlier that day, Castillo had slow cooked a pot of black beans with laurel, onions, garlic, and local jalapeños. She now slid the pot nearer the flames. When the beans came to a boil, she added a few cups of cooked rice.

Then she spooned lime-soaked corn kernels from a galvanized steel pail into a hand grinder and cranked out a pile of corn dough—or masa, as she called it. She patted out tortillas and roasted them over the open fire. On a crude iron griddle, she melted a dollop of lard and fried some eggs. Finally she cut paper-thin slices of fresh cheese—an impressive feat given her poor eyesight. I later learned she could barely see the cheese, much less her fingers.

In a half hour, she presented us with lunch—small portions of *gallo pinto,* the iconic Costa Rican rice-and-bean dish, garnished with cheese and cilantro, corn tortillas, and one egg on a small plate. The serving looked huge, but it amounted to about half of what you'd get if you ordered the breakfast special at your local diner.

"Food gives life!" she shouted, and sat us down to eat.

Like most of the region's centenarians, Castillo has lived a hard life. The Nicoya Peninsula was largely cut off from progress until the last couple of decades. Only rough dirt roads—mud roads in the rainy season—etched the hilly terrain. For most of her life, Castillo ran her parents' small boardinghouse for itinerant *sabaneros,* the region's leathery cowboys.

Aside from beans and tortillas, she raises or grows much of her own food in her garden—or gathers it from nearby fruit trees. Her strong belief in

God helped her raise five children—two of whom are great-grandfathers now—and helped her survive the violent death of one of them. Yet despite all these hardships, she gets up each morning, puts on a bright pink dress and party beads, sweeps off her deck, and greets daily visitors with a gleeful "God blesses us."

The people of Nicoya descend mostly from the Chorotega. But they are also genetically influenced by Spanish colonists and freed African slaves. In the past they died largely of regional diseases such as malaria, dysentery, diarrhea, and dengue, which was menacingly dubbed "broken bone disease." During the 1980s the dry forests, dominated by the enormous, regally tufted *guanacaste* trees, was a refuge for the Contras, the U.S.-funded counterrevolutionaries who at the time were mounting armed resistance to Nicaragua's communist Sandinistas.

Today middle-aged people here—especially men—reach a healthy, vital age of 90 at rates up to 2.5 times greater than those in the United States. In other words, residents here elude heart disease, many types of cancer, and diabetes better than Americans by an order of magnitude. And they spend about one-fifteenth of what the United States spends on health care. How do they do it?

My colleagues, demographers Michel Poulain and Luis Rosero-Bixby of the University of Costa Rica, and I conducted two expeditions here to solve this mystery. Together we concluded that the Nicoyans' secret lies partly in their strong faith community, in their deep social networks, and their habit of doing regular, low-intensity physical activity. They also benefited from a healthy dose of vitamin D from sunlight and extra calcium in their water—more, in fact, than anywhere else in the country. The combination may lead to stronger bones and fewer fatal falls for seniors. Diet plays a big role too.

THE NICOYAN PANTRY OF THE PAST

From my interviews with Castillo and some 40 other Costa Rican centenarians, I knew what the typical Nicoyan kitchen held. The lunch she served me pretty much represented what people had been eating here for at least the past century. But I had another source to lean on. In preparing for one trip, I'd found a 1957 report entitled *Nicoya: A Cultural Geography*, written by a young Berkeley anthropologist named Phillip Wagner. In it, he described a day in the life of an average Nicoyan—50 years ago:

> The day of the country people begins before sunrise, when the women rise to prepare coffee. The family meets about dawn to take a cup of black coffee, or coffee with milk, heavily sweetened, and perhaps to eat a cold tortilla. The time from dawn to eight o'clock is for chores and beginning the day's work. At eight there may be a complete breakfast with rice and beans and eggs. In seasons of heavy work the men take with them to the fields tortillas with gallo pinto (rice and beans fried in pork fat). Work may end on very hot days at twelve, or at two in the afternoon. The workers come home from the fields or the woods and wait about an hour for their meal. The midday meal often begins with a pot of soup in which there are a few bits of meat, fat, boiled plantains, tesquisque [taro] or yuca, and perhaps a few greens. After the soup come rice and beans, usually accompanied by fried eggs. On occasion there may also be some vegetable: pipian or ayote *(Cucurbita moschata)* or calabaza [both types of squash], cabbage, the flower of pinuela [a wild plant related to pineapple] or some other wild product. Meat sometimes appears on even the poorest table, and there is usually cuajada, a milk curd. Tortillas come with this meal and afterward the men sip heavily sweetened black coffee, made from local berries or from the mashed seeds of nanju *(Hibiscus esculentus)*. The evening meal is simpler, since the custom is to spend the afternoon in idleness and appetites are less hearty. Rice and beans, tortillas and perhaps eggs are served just at dusk.

Wagner also made detailed sketches of gardens, showing more than 40 different edible plant species, highlighting the yucca, taro, papaya, yam, guava, cashew, and banana as mainstays of the local diet. Nicoyans also ate a wide variety of forest fruits not likely to show up at your local grocery store, such as *caimito*—the sweet, purple star apple, very high in antioxidants—and *papaturro,* also known as *coccoloba,* or sea grapes. For more detail, I contacted Xinia Fernández at the University of Costa Rica's School of Nutrition, who provided me with three dietary evaluations, as they were called, from 1969, 1978, and 1982. Nutritionists visited families daily to help them record their dietary intake and weighed food when possible—a labor-intensive and expensive process that yielded good insights.

According to these surveys, the Nicoyan diet was high in carbohydrates—about 68 percent, a level matched only by the Okinawan diet and much higher than the average American diet. Their main carbohydrate sources were rice, maize, and beans. Fat was just over 20 percent and protein was about 10 percent, accounting for the other 30 percent of their daily diet. All told, the average person in the Chorotega region consumed about 1,800 calories a day.

A few characteristics of Nicoya's diet stood out. Like residents of most other Blue Zones, people here ate a low-calorie, low-fat, plant-based diet rich in legumes. Traditionally, they lived mostly off beans, corn tortillas, and huge quantities of tropical fruits. Sweet lemon, sweet orange *(Citrus sinensis),* and a banana variety called *cuadrado* have been the most common fruits throughout most of the year in Nicoya.

The big secret of the Nicoyan diet was the "three sisters" of Mesoamerican agriculture: beans, corn, and squash. Since at least 5000 B.C. Mesoamericans living in and around modern-day Guatemala and Mexico have been cultivating beans, squash, and corn in fields called milpas, a brilliant agricultural system in which each crop benefits from the others. The squash provide ground cover to hold in moisture. The cornstalks grow high and the bean vines twine up them. The bean plants fix nitrogen as a fertilizer in the soil.

An almost perfect agricultural cycle, the resulting crops, consumed in combination, amount to an almost perfect food combination for human sustenance as well. A combination of cooked beans and squash, eaten with corn tortillas, is rich in complex carbohydrates, protein, calcium, and niacin. It naturally helps reduce bad cholesterol and increase good cholesterol. Nutritionist Leonardo Mata, whom I interviewed in Costa Rica's capital, San José, told me he thought the most significant component of the Nicoyan diet was how they prepared their corn. To prepare the dough that Nicoyans call *maize nixquezado,* they soak whole corn kernels in calcium hydroxide, or lime and water, which infuses the grain with 7.5 times more calcium and unlocks certain amino acids otherwise unavailable in the corn. Mata has been studying cultures throughout Central America that prepare corn the same way, and he claims that the people who consume it regularly never get rickets and rarely suffer the bone fractures and broken hips that often lead to premature death in older people.

During the past 50 years, white rice has largely replaced squash as a daily staple in Nicoya. Although lower in fiber and nutrients than

Typical Daily Diet of Rural Costa Ricans, mid-1960s
(Percentage of daily intake in grams)

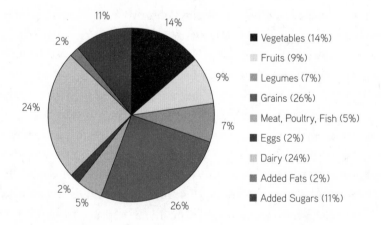

- Vegetables (14%)
- Fruits (9%)
- Legumes (7%)
- Grains (26%)
- Meat, Poultry, Fish (5%)
- Eggs (2%)
- Dairy (24%)
- Added Fats (2%)
- Added Sugars (11%)

Source: Flores and INCAP and ICNND.

In the traditional Nicoyan diet, about 80 percent of daily calories came from carbohydrates, with the remaining 20 percent coming from proteins and fats in about equal measure.

and soluble fiber. They are nearly a staple food in Nicoya and the most common. The sweet varieties are picked fresh, peeled, and eaten—the go-to snack. Some types do not sweeten as they ripen. The plantain, for instance, must be boiled or fried and is served like a potato.

PEJIVALLES (PEACH PALMS) Clusters of this small, orange, oval fruit dangle from palm trees throughout Central America. A staple food for Costa Rica's indigenous people yet rarely if ever seen for sale in the United States, it is especially high in vitamins A and C. Traditionally the fruit was stewed in salted water and served with salt or honey. One prominent Costa Rican researcher also believes that *pejivalles* may interact with a bacterium *(Helicobacter pylori)* that is closely associated with stomach cancer. Peach palms in their diet may, therefore, explain why Nicoyans have the lowest rates of stomach cancer in Costa Rica.

For recipes from Nicoya, see pages 287–297.

PART TWO

Making
an American
Blue Zone

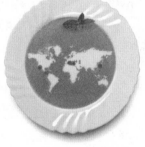

D ID YOU NOTICE THAT NONE OF THE INDIVIDUALS we met in part 1—Athina Mazari, Gozei Shinzato, the Melis family, Ellsworth Wareham, or Panchita Castillo—ever willed themselves to eat the right foods? They never read labels, counted calories, weighed their protein, or signed up for Weight Watchers. Yet they all ate a nearly perfect diet *without thinking about it.*

How did they do it? The surprisingly simple answer: They lived in environments that encouraged healthy eating. Fresh fruits and vegetables were affordable and readily available year-round. Sodas, chips, sweets, and burgers—foods they might like to eat too, just as we do—were hard to find. Their neighborhoods weren't a forest of advertising for junk foods they might crave. Their homes were set up in a way that made it easy for them to prepare plant-based foods for the table, and they had time-honored recipes to make them taste good. Their faith-based organizations and social networks supported selecting, preparing, and eating the right kinds of foods. Doing things that helped them maintain a healthy weight, stay connected, and keep physically active weren't just choices—they represented a shared way of life.

Compare that to the experience of the typical American. According to Brian Wansink of Cornell University, a co-director of the Blue Zones Project, the average American makes about 200 food decisions a day. But as Wansink points out, most of us are aware of only about 30 of them. The rest fall into the category of what he calls "mindless" behavior. Consider what happens at lunch. You've resolved to order a light lunch but now that you see the buffalo wing appetizers on the menu, they sound kind of good. And as you scan the list of salads for a healthy choice, your colleague orders the Reuben and fries and you blurt, "I'll have the same"—though you're not sure why. Do you really want to put ketchup and more salt on those fries? And how about that free refill on your soda? Then there's dessert . . .

In the Blue Zones, on the other hand, food and lifestyle decisions flowed from the environment, and their surroundings provided them with only healthy choices. Castillo didn't have a microwave. Ellsworth ate at home so he could control what he consumed. Shinzato cooked mostly what grew in her garden. The Melis family ate lunches with their kin. And Mazari relied on the time-honored recipes of her ancestors.

To understand what we eat—and why, in modern America, we eat too many of the wrong foods and too much overall—we need to look beyond ourselves and our personal habits. We need to become aware of the influence of the environment: that radius of 20 miles or so from our homes where we shop, work, walk or drive, attend school, eat at restaurants, and spend most of our lives. Here, within this zone, is where we're constantly nudged into healthy or unhealthy choices, based on the norms and habits of the people around us, the laws and ordinances of our community, and the decisions that have been made, conscious or not, about all the features that make it a healthy place to live—or not.

Once we began to understand how the environments of the Blue Zones had made them especially healthy places to live, we started to imagine how to create Blue Zones in America. Could an American community make certain changes, adopting some of the same pathways to longevity that work so well elsewhere in the world? For the past six years, that has been my mission.

In the chapters that follow, we'll visit several remarkable communities whose successes suggest that a Blue Zones solution can work for anyone, any town. We'll start with a region in rural Finland that convinced me it could be done and set our Blue Zones makeover project in motion. We'll drop in on a Minnesota prairie town that shed more than two tons of weight in a single year. We'll get to know three Los Angeles municipalities that reduced obesity by 14 percent. We'll spend time in Iowa farm communities where cholesterol levels have dropped 4 percent, while volunteerism has increased by 10 percent, and business leaders have replaced sit-down meetings with walking ones.

None of these communities relied on draconian diets or herculean discipline to achieve their goals. Instead, they identified dozens of small steps to create a healthier environment that led to a healthy swarm of grassroots initiatives. The cumulative effect of these positive nudges was a long-lasting change—one with a far greater impact than any individual's willpower or discipline could ever have.

CHAPTER SIX

❧

Finland's Miracle Makeover

I T WAS A COLD SUMMER AFTERNOON and I sat in a warm Helsinki office in Finland's National Institute for Health and Welfare across from Pekka Puska. He didn't look like the renegade I imagined. His outfit was vintage bureaucratic chic: polyester khakis, white, short-sleeved shirt, a crooked brown tie, sensible shoes, and a stainless-steel Citizen watch. But his clear blue eyes and boyish good looks reminded me of an older Steve McQueen. Diplomas, awards, and framed photographs of public health legends adorned his office walls. Four decades ago, Puska, now 68, pioneered a strategy that turned around the lives of more than 170,000 Finns, a population that was suffering from the highest rate of heart disease in the world. Though he didn't know it then, he essentially manufactured a Blue Zone in Scandinavia. And he did it by breaking all of the established rules of public health.

"Let me tell you a story," Puska began, leaning forward and resting both of his elbows on the table where we sat. "There were two rival fire brigades, a volunteer one and the official one. A fire broke out, and, for some reason, the volunteer brigade got there first and extinguished the fire. When the official brigade came later, they said it was incorrectly extinguished."

He paused. "You get my point, right?" he said, blue eyes glinting and still reveling in the revolutionary way he had changed public health.

Back in 1968 Puska had been a firebrand, president of the National Student Union while at the University of Turku, where he'd fought for student rights. "These were turbulent times in Europe," he recalled. "There was a feeling we could change the world."

After graduation, the young activist landed a job with the Department of Public Health. At about the same time, results were coming in from national and international statistics. They pointed to one region of Finland—North Karelia, a New Jersey–size region of boreal forests in the far eastern part of the country—as having particularly severe health problems. For years, as good, compliant Finns, the North Karelians had submitted to these surveys and tests without question. But when they discovered that their population was distinguished by the highest rate of heart disease in the world, they became indignant. The government responded by approving a small grant, tapping Puska, then 27, with a medical degree and a master's in social sciences, to lead a five-year pilot project in the region.

"I wasn't hired because I was good," Puska said, recalling what his boss told him many years later. "I was hired because I was young, and he knew it was going to take decades to figure out the problem."

With his grassroots organizing background, Puska and his team took an approach different from the traditional top-down government effort. Beginning in 1972, he worked with local health care systems and community organizations to disseminate a new message, and in the long run, they nudged the people of North Karelia into adopting a low-fat, high-vegetable diet. Among many other initiatives, Finnish scientists developed a type of rapeseed (canola) that would grow in Finland's boreal climate and marketed its oil as a butter replacement. They showed housewives how they could make traditional meals with vegetables as well as meat.

By the end of the five-year project they were seeing impressive results. North Karelia reduced the heart attack death rate among middle-aged men by 25 percent. Lung cancer deaths in the same group fell by 10 percent, largely because of a dramatic reduction in smoking. Since then, the reduction in lung cancer mortality has been 20 percent. Mortality from all cancers dropped by 10 percent. The rest of Finland has followed the example of North Karelia and has also seen big improvements in these categories. Life expectancy of Finnish males in general has jumped by nearly ten years in these last three decades.

As a result of his successes, Puska went on to become the head of the National Institute for Health and Welfare in Finland and president of the World Health Federation. I think of him as the Che Guevara of public health initiatives. The popular press refers to the North Karelia Project as "The Miracle Up North." To date it's never been replicated—though we're giving it a good try with our Blue Zones community makeovers.

A FORMULA FOR CHANGE

What was it about Puska's campaign in North Karelia that made it so effective? Could I learn anything from his team's strategies to bring similar health benefits to American communities? These were the questions on my mind as I dug deeper into his story.

Dotted with 450 lakes and several hundred villages, North Karelia tucks into a crook of Finland's border with Russia. Many of the taciturn, hard-working people who live there—descendants of reindeer herders—are farmers and lumberjacks, so quintessentially Finnish that they are often called the most Finnish of Finns.

Before World War II, most North Karelians lived off the land, picking berries, hunting game, and fishing for perch, pike, smelt, and lake salmon. Besides the occasional bear mauling, their main health concerns were tuberculosis, infectious diseases, and death at childbirth. But after the war, hospital beds started filling up with victims of heart disease. Otherwise healthy men in their 30s and 40s were dropping dead from heart attacks. It wasn't bad luck that was killing them—it was smoking and their diet.

During the war, when food was scarce, families in North Karelia had survived on rye bread, potatoes, and meat. That changed dramatically after the war, when veterans, as part of their compensation, were given small plots of land. Most of these veterans possessed little or no agricultural training, but it was easy enough for them to clear the land, buy a few pigs and dairy cows, and begin to support their families. That set the stage for what experts described as the world's deadliest diet.

Take a half-starved population with a taste for fat and give them an abundance of pigs and dairy cows, and you've got a recipe for trouble. Butter soon made its way into almost every meal: butter-fried potatoes, buttered bread, tall glasses of full-cream milk at every meal, fried pork or meat stew for dinner, chased with buttered bread and milk. Vegetables were considered food for the animals. And dairy wasn't just a source of calories, it was a source of regional pride. Yet it was taking a terrible toll.

Alarmed by this epidemic of heart disease, a Finnish professor named Martti Karvonen came to the United States in 1954 in search of possible solutions. One of the experts he consulted was Ancel Keys, a dietary researcher at the University of Minnesota in Minneapolis whom he'd met a few years before in Europe at a meeting of the Food and Agriculture Organization (FAO) of the United Nations. Keys had been promoting his hypothesis—controversial at the time and still attacked by some today—about the association between eating animal products and heart disease. Karvonen and Keys decided to join forces.

In what would become known as the Seven Countries Study, Karvonen, Keys, and their colleagues recruited groups of middle-aged men for a long-term project not only in Finland but also in the United States, Japan, Italy, the Netherlands, Greece, and Yugoslavia. Each subject in the study was asked questions about his diet and given a battery of physical tests. Then, at five-year intervals, the study checked in on him again. A pattern soon emerged: The farther north the men lived, the more dietary fat they tended to consume (mostly from meat and dairy). In Greece and Italy, where people ate mostly a plant-based diet, men were largely free of heart disease—an observation that eventually informed our understanding of the value of the traditional Mediterranean diet. (Keys has been criticized for omitting government data on diet and heart disease from certain countries that he compared early on. But Keys had good reason to leave out the data: Death certificates were undependable, and World War II had disrupted the food supply in those countries. Moreover, in the seven countries study he had gone on to measure people directly and find a higher heart attack risk where they ate a higher proportion of animal foods.) In places like North Karelia (the study's northern extreme), conversely, men were *30 times* more likely to die of heart attacks than in places like Crete. In fact, North Karelian men on average were dying ten years earlier than their counterparts in the south. It got so bad that, by 1972, North Karelian men achieved the dubious distinction of having the highest rate of heart disease in the world.

"The researchers would come here year after year, ask us questions, poke us with needles, and tell us we were the most unhealthy people in the world," recalled Esa Timonen, the former governor of the region. "At a certain point we said, 'Enough!'"

A NEW APPROACH

At the time, the causes of heart disease were still a mystery; doctors didn't agree on what caused it, never mind how to cure it. So the first thing Puska did when he arrived in Joensuu, North Karelia's capital, was to organize an idealistic young team to tackle the problem. They started by using essentially the same strategy that health officials had used to fight infectious diseases like tuberculosis or polio. They set up surveys to capture people's health information. They identified the sick or the most-likely-to-get-sick, and then came up with prescriptions to help the highest-risk people stay healthier. After that, the team gave out health information and set targets for the community to achieve in their efforts to lower heart disease. The problem, they soon realized, was that instead of a vaccination or an antibiotic to cure heart disease, the best medicine was avoiding many of the foods central to North Karelian culture. They printed up leaflets and posters, imploring people to consume less fat and salt and to eat more vegetables. But these Finns loved their bread, butter, and fried pork. How could you break such habits?

"I could see the whole system needed to change," Puska said. "The food industry, restaurants, cafeterias, and supermarkets—from the bottom up." He started by consulting Geoffrey Rose, a British epidemiologist who believed that it was more cost-effective to prevent disease than to cure it. In Rose's opinion, hospitals and doctors could no more solve the problem of general ill health than famine relief could solve the problem of world hunger. He was the first to show using epidemiological data that the number of people who died of heart disease was directly proportional to the average blood pressure levels of the whole population. He also calculated that for every percentage point you lowered cholesterol in a population, you lowered heart disease by two points. Whether you lived a short sick life or a long healthy one, Rose argued, was a function of the population you belonged to more than the quality of your doctor or hospital care. Puska took this lesson to heart, realizing that the only way to cure North Karelia of heart disease was to change the local culture.

Puska and his team approached the Martha Organization, a powerful women's organization with several local clubs, to help spread the word. Together, Puska and the clubs hatched the idea of holding afternoon "longevity parties," where a member of Puska's team would give a short talk about the connection between saturated fat and heart attacks. They gave the women a recipe book that added vegetables to traditional North Karelian dishes and cooked and served them. North Karelian stew, for instance, typically had only three main ingredients—water, fatty pork, and salt—but the team replaced some of the pork with rutabagas, potatoes, and carrots. The women liked the new version of the dish, which they named Puska's stew. By showing these farm wives how to cook plant-based meals that tasted good, Puska had found a way to disseminate the health message better than any leaflet could.

Puska, inspired by a former professor, Everett Rogers, who came up with the idea of "opinion leaders," next went from village to village recruiting "lay ambassadors." Believing that the best way to spark cultural change was from the bottom up, he recruited some 1,500 people, usually women who were already involved in other civic organizations. He gave each ambassador an identification card, taught them simple messages about reducing salt and fat consumption (and how to quit smoking), and encouraged them to talk to their friends.

Just Move Home

During my stay in North Karelia, I hired Elisa Korpelainen, the daughter of one of the North Karelia Project's leaders, as a translator. She set up meetings for me, translated conversations, drove me to meetings, and offered insight into the local culture. Though only 20, Korpelainen possessed a maturity you wouldn't expect from an American of the same age. I once asked her if she knew any Finnish jokes. She couldn't think of any. "We're pretty serious people here," she said without a trace of self-consciousness. When I asked if Finns ever just sat around and acted sullen for fun, she frowned at me.

Korpelainen had recently returned from a stay in Cork, Ireland, where she'd taken a job as a kennel and stable hand trainer. It had been a rigorous 11 months, she said, working from morning to night cleaning kennels, minding the stables, and riding horses. Despite that, she'd gained eight pounds in Ireland by eating a standard modern diet of fast food, frozen dinners, and cookies with tea. "I was carrying a little extra weight when I got back home," she confessed.

Tall and slender, Korpelainen had a roundish face with slate blue eyes that were framed by shoulder-length blond hair. She often wore long gauzy scarves that she coiled around her neck. Somehow, during the three months since she'd returned to North Karelia, she'd lost all of those pounds, she said. I asked if she went on a diet or if she'd started working out.

"No, I actually work less than I did in Ireland," she said.

"Then what did you do to lose all that weight?"

"Nothing," she replied blankly. "I just moved home."

His small, underfunded staff tried everything they could think of to infiltrate the community. Puska spoke relentlessly at churches, community centers, and schools. He became the face of this new health movement, constantly recruiting people to the cause. (One of his mentors once told him that the only way to succeed in prevention is to "push, push, push." His English-speaking friends later joked, "Now we know why your name is Puska!") Soon the message about replacing saturated fat with fruits and vegetables began to resonate with the people. They were starting to make a difference.

Next Puska started to lobby food producers. You could have the world's best program to educate people about how to eat healthier, he figured, but if they weren't able to obtain healthy ingredients, then what good was it? The regional sausage company, for example, loaded its products with pork fat and salt. Traditional breads were laced with butter. Karelian cows, developed from breeds known as Finncattle, produced some of the fattiest milk in the world, and dairy subsidies rewarded high fat content.

At first, none of the businesses was interested in formulating healthier versions of their products. Why should they risk profits? In fact, the powerful dairy industry fought back, taking out ads bashing the project. But the ads backfired, because they sparked a public debate, waking up many people to the connection between dairy fat and heart disease.

North Karelians were also realizing that they needed to eat more fruits, but common fruits such as oranges or melons were expensive: They had to be imported from southern Europe, and they played no part in the Karelians' traditional diet. Puska saw a homegrown solution: berries.

During the summer, blueberries, raspberries, and lingonberries grew abundantly in the region, and North Karelians loved them. But they ate them only in the late summer, during the short berry season. So Puska's team supported the establishment of cooperatives and businesses to freeze, process, and distribute berries. They convinced local dairy farmers to apportion some of their pastureland to grow berries and convinced grocers to stock frozen berries. As soon as berries became available year-round, fruit consumption soared.

After five years, Puska's project was producing impressive numbers. North Karelians saw their average cholesterol numbers drop by 6 percent and their average blood pressure drop 4 percent for men and 7 percent for women. Even so, some academics criticized Puska because they said it

The Sausage Maker

The nutrition campaign in North Karelia got a break when the team met Aare Halonen, a local sausage maker. As it happened, Halonen had recently suffered a heart attack and was receptive to the team's health message. They persuaded him to reformulate some of his products by replacing a portion of the pork fat in his sausages with mushrooms, which happened to be a cheap local filler. Halonen did it gradually, over a period of months, and the result was a product with good flavor but significantly lower fat and salt content. The timing turned out to be good. As local customers began to embrace the low-fat message, sales of Halonen's new sausages began to soar.

Pekka Puska's project scored a similar success with local bakeries, convincing them to lower sodium content and replace butter with vegetable oil as a shortening. "Consumers didn't even know the difference," Puska said. They were eating healthier without even trying.

was impossible to pinpoint exactly what had caused the improving numbers. Was it the drop in meat consumption? The rise in vegetable and fruit consumption? A rising health awareness among the general public? His medical colleagues ridiculed the project, calling it "shotgun medicine." But as it turns out, Puska's strategy worked: He may have fired a shotgun, but he unleashed a healthy blast of silver buckshot that saved lives.

STRATEGIC LESSONS

Not long ago, I visited North Karelia to see how this miracle had transformed people's lives. Boarding a train in Helsinki, I traveled 250 miles north, passing through boreal forests and pea green fields that swooped and curved like curlicues on a paisley shirt. Homesteads dotted the landscape—cozy, compact houses painted bright red or burnt yellow, with medieval-looking plank barns out back. When I arrived in Joensuu, the sun was arcing low over the Scandinavian sky. A brassy light illuminated the city's birch-lined streets, lakefront houses, and Lutheran churches.

I found the headquarters of the North Karelia Project on the sixth floor of a brick building that fronted the town plaza. It was a cramped jumble of four small offices furnished with Ikea-style desks and lined with 30 years of records in neat file folders. There, I met Vesa Korpelainen, a tall, serious man with sandy brown hair, blue jeans, and a red-checkered shirt. Since 1986 he'd been Puska's man on the ground in North Karelia. He told me how he motivated his team.

"We have two slogans that drive our work," he said. "'Face-to-face communication' and 'common interest.' It's extremely important to get people involved. That means you have to be honest. You have to work with people—on the same level." He described his team's daily activities as "meetings, meetings, meetings," and he attributed their success to a "relentless, congenial nudging" rather than any heroic initiatives.

As I listened to Korpelainen, the various pieces of the North Karelia campaign began to come together in my mind. Partly through trial and error, but also through tremendous dedication and persistence, Puska and his team had developed a winning strategy. If I was looking for a model for how to manufacture a Blue Zone in America, I needed to absorb the principles of their work.

To show me how these strategies had been put into practice in the capital, Korpelainen took me on a walking tour of Joensuu. We first visited a grocery store, where he pointed out products inspired by the project: rows of healthy butter substitutes and candies sweetened with xylitol, a natural sweetener made from birch sap. In an open market we saw row after row of berry and wild mushroom vendors. There were only two holdouts from the old dietary regime: One vendor sold butter-fried smelt; another offered pocket pastries filled with rice porridge and about a half stick of butter each. After that we breezed through a restaurant and saw the prominent salad bar. Soft drinks were served in small glasses and customers paid for refills.

I was eager to meet some of the people Puska had tapped as ambassadors. I had heard that they tended to weigh less and have lower health care costs

Lessons Learned From North Karelia

- **FOCUS ON THE ECOLOGY OF HEALTH** Pekka Puska's team didn't waste anybody's time by lecturing them about individual responsibility. Instead, they put their resources into making long-lasting changes to the local *environment*.
- **THINK OPERATING SYSTEM, NOT PROGRAM** The team developed a nimble, flexible approach that allowed them to innovate constantly.
- **WORK WITH LOCAL HEALTH SYSTEMS** People listen to their doctors and nurses. The team recruited local health professionals to help disseminate the message.
- **PUSH, PUSH, PUSH** Working with "boots in the mud" was one of the North Karelia team's mantras. They succeeded by relentless, congenial gnawing at the problem rather than heroic initiatives.
- **FIND A CHARISMATIC LEADER** People like to identify a movement with individuals, and North Karelia found its leader in Puska.
- **COMMUNITY OWNERSHIP** The leadership and population of North Karelia was ready for a change. That made the work of the team easier, because they were responding to a plea from the community for help with heart disease.
- **BOTTOM UP, TOP DOWN** The project team spent time and resources at the grassroots level to help people realize that their problem was diet. Then they harnessed that understanding to change food policy and the food system from the top down. The heavy lifting was done by the people themselves, making the connections between the two.
- **MEASURE, MEASURE, MEASURE** The team vigilantly measured the population's lifestyle risk factors, including smoking and other health factors, at the beginning, middle, and end of the project to track progress and be able to prove the strategy worked.
- **START SMALL, GO BIG** Once North Karelia proved that this approach worked, Finland's national health system instituted an effective countrywide preventive program, following a similar model.

than non-volunteers of the same age. First I met 78-year-old Pentti Seutu, who confirmed that image. When I arrived at his home, Seutu was ripping through a pile of logs with a chain saw. Inside, his wife had prepared a dinner of vegetable casserole with lingonberry jam, a mushroom salad, fresh garden vegetables—cucumbers, lettuce, tomatoes—and two types of heavy rye breads. I asked Seutu why he'd volunteered for the project. "I like the feeling of giving back," he said. "Besides, there's not much else to do up here during the long months and the short days of winter."

Outside of Joensuu, I met Mauno and Helka Lempinen in their snug cottage set in an apple orchard. Mauno, another wood cutter in his late 90s, was splitting wood when I arrived. The couple invited me inside, where we sat in a sunroom with warm birch floors covered by pastel carpets Helka had woven. The couple had come to North Karelia in 1973, when Mauno took a job as school principal. He soon adopted the local traditions and, like everybody else, started his day with buttered bread and coffee, lunched on cold cut sandwiches, and dined on pork stew. Vegetables were almost nonexistent as a part of their meals, he said. "People here thought of them as curiosities."

In 1983 Mauno suffered a heart attack. The couple went into great detail describing to me how he panted "like he was giving birth" and the trauma it caused their three children who witnessed it. Emergency open-heart surgery saved his life. I asked how that had altered their lifestyle, expecting a long list of healthy adjustments.

"Oh, we didn't change anything." Helka said.

Puzzled, I asked about their normal diet today. "Well, for breakfast I had porridge with fruit. Lunch was vegetable soup with homemade rye bread," Helka responded. "Dinner will be stew with potatoes and carrots and a little bit of meat, along with cucumber and lettuce salad."

What then, I asked, prompted them to change the diet?

"We never changed our diet," they insisted.

Wait a minute, I said, and flipped through my notes to read them the butter-and-pork pre–heart attack menu they'd described to me earlier.

"Well, I guess we did change our diet," Helka said after a long pause. When I asked why, they looked down and thought hard. They had no idea. "It just happened," Mauno said finally. "But I guess it saved my life." It occurred to me that herein lay the true miracle of North Karelia. An entire population, just like this couple, had changed their lifestyle *without realizing it.*

There it was, I thought: the key to Puska's strategy. The North Karelia campaign had tackled the region's health problem from so many different directions, its reforms were all but invisible. In Sardinia or Okinawa, centuries of cultural evolution had led to a lifestyle of long life, but here was a place that had *manufactured* a Blue Zone and given its population a ten-year bump in longevity. And they had done so without massive health care spending.

They'd simply changed their environment.

I had found my example. A rural community in far-flung Finland had made deliberate decisions, changed their diet and eating habits, adapted their traditions, and improved their health. But a small Finnish region is one thing—could this sort of transformation take place in 21st-century America?

MEASURES OF SUCCESS IN NORTH KARELIA

- When the North Karelia Project began, more than half of all men in the region smoked. Today only 20 percent do.
- In a region of dairy farms, the proportion of residents consuming high-fat milk has dropped from about 70 percent to less than 10 percent.
- About 60 percent of households now cook mainly with vegetable oil.
- Less than 5 percent of households still use butter on bread, compared to about 84 percent in 1972.
- Overall salt intake has fallen by about 20 percent.
- Vegetable consumption has increased threefold.
- The average cholesterol level has dropped by 20 percent.
- The heart disease death rate among working-age men has fallen by 85 percent.

CHAPTER SEVEN

❧

The Minnesota Experiment

I HAD THE ANSWER TO MY QUESTION—or so I thought. As Pekka Puska and his team had so dramatically shown in Finland, it was indeed possible to take an unhealthy population and transform it into a healthy one. Individuals and families didn't have to be born inside a Blue Zone to benefit from Blue Zones principles. With the right help, they could apply those same principles to create a Blue Zone right where they lived. Puska had proven that in North Karelia. But could it be done here in the United States? I still wasn't sure. A lot depended on a small group of decision-makers in a little town in southern Minnesota.

They were all there in the conference room: the mayor, city manager, superintendent of schools, head of public health, president of the chamber of commerce, and respected business leaders—the movers and shakers in the town of Albert Lea, Minnesota. They were gathered on this September morning in 2008 to hear why I thought they should ignite a Blue Zones revolution in their quiet community.

It was simple, I told them. Our nation was heading in the wrong direction with our health and eating habits. We spent almost a trillion dollars a year on preventable diseases but devoted only 3 percent of our health care budget to prevention. The vast majority of our money went for treating illnesses that we could avoid, such as coronary heart disease, diabetes, and cancer. Meanwhile, two-thirds of us were obese or overweight. Everybody knew we were on the wrong track, but nobody seemed to be able to turn us around.

"That's why I've come to Albert Lea," I said. "Along with a few members of my team, I'm visiting a handful of towns in Minnesota to see if one might be a good choice for a unique pilot project. We're looking for a community that isn't too big or too small, too healthy or too unhealthy, to work with us on an experiment to change a town's whole ecosystem."

"I'll tell you exactly how we're going to do it," I said. "We're going to focus on a 20-mile radius around your homes and jobs. That's where your supermarkets, favorite restaurants, and school cafeterias are located. Is it easy to walk downtown? Are parks clean and attractive? Are you allowed to smoke in public places? What about schools and workplaces: Are soda pops and salty snacks the only foods that are cheap and easily available? Instead of relying on individual responsibility, an approach that hasn't worked, we're going to work on your surroundings."

We're also going to work on your social ecosystem, I said—people's connections, network of friends and associates, sense of belonging. "Research has shown that if your three best friends are obese, there's a 50 percent greater chance that you'll be overweight too."

I told them we were partnering with AARP, which was providing generous financial support, and that we had significant interest from national media outlets like ABC and USA Today. "If this sounds like something you'd like to try in Albert Lea," I said, "we'd like you to apply to be the first Blue Zones city."

I sat down and waited for their response. Silence. I could hear the ticking of a clock. As I glanced around the table, I saw skeptical expressions. Maybe I hadn't explained the plan as well as I could have? Maybe it was too much to ask of a small midwestern town. Maybe they thought I was just another guy with a crazy idea. The moment seemed to last forever.

Then a voice broke the silence. It was Bob Graham, the longtime town planner. If anybody knew and loved the place, it was Graham. "This is exactly what Albert Lea needs," he said. "We need to do this."

Then another person spoke up. "It wouldn't be hard to get volunteers," she said. They had lists from other recent collaborations.

"Well, how would you get employers on board?" someone asked.

"And what about seniors? How can we get them involved?"

Soon the group was kicking around ideas to get the project rolling. It looked like the revolution might happen after all.

THE GOOD NEWS AND THE BAD

Things didn't seem as positive a few months before. I'd been talking to Robert L. Kane, a professor at the University of Minnesota School of Public Health, about ways to apply the lessons I'd learned from the Blue Zones to people here in the United States. As a good friend, he'd been giving me a reality check.

Kane, a leading expert on aging, had been a key source when I was writing *The Blue Zones*. If people wanted to live longer, he told me, the most important things they could do, after giving up smoking, would be to eat moderately, exercise regularly, maintain friendships, and pursue an interest that makes life meaningful. But what if individuals found it too difficult to stick with such things on their own, Kane was asking. "You have to make these things a habit that people do for a long time, or they don't work," he warned.

That's where North Karelia came in. What if we did something similar here in the United States by weaving Blue Zones principles into every aspect of a community—from restaurants and businesses to schools and homes?

I knew I wasn't the first to think of community-wide health transformation in America. In fact, a number of "noninfectious disease community interventions," as Kane called them, had been tried. One of the largest had been organized a few decades ago at his own School of Public Health. With a multimillion-dollar grant from the National Institutes of Health (NIH), researchers in 1980 had launched the Minnesota Heart Health Program in six towns near Minneapolis, three experimental and three control groups. The aim was to see if a population-based approach—including activities at schools, workplaces, and restaurants—could reduce cardiovascular diseases. But after six years of trying, the results were disappointing. Although all groups improved, researchers had found no difference between the towns where actions had been taken and the control cities—those where nothing had been done.

Two other large NIH studies, the Stanford Five-City Project and the Pawtucket Heart Health Program, had ended the same way. As a result, the government had stopped funding large-scale community experiments, Kane said. "There was this wave of big social experiments a generation ago, but not much since then." I knew he was right, but I couldn't let go of the idea that creating Blue Zones in the United States was possible.

Whether convinced or not, Kane introduced me to John Finnegan, dean of the university's School of Public Health, who invited me to address a faculty meeting in the summer of 2008. When I arrived, I was greeted by 15 experts in public health and epidemiology who'd been involved in community trials. We talked about what Puska had done in Finland, and I gave them a brief presentation with slides that mapped out my vision of how a Blue Zones makeover of an American city could be just as effective. I told them that, to me, the key to changing a community's health was to target its environment rather than individual behaviors. Then we had a free-flowing conversation for two hours or so.

"What about its size?" I asked them. If we were to organize a community makeover, how big should the town be?

Robert W. Jeffery, an expert in community health, diet, and obesity, suggested the perfect size might be a population between 15,000 and 20,000.

Then somebody else said, "You should pick a town close enough to the Twin Cities that you and your team can travel back and forth inexpensively." She suggested we only consider towns within a 90-mile radius.

Meanwhile, Kane kept playing the skeptic. He asked how we would assess our success, and suggested that we measure the blood pressure and cholesterol levels of the entire community before and after. That would give us the best scientific data, but the cost of such tests would have exhausted our entire budget.

"How are you going to get people to take part?" someone asked. "How are you going to get them to stick with the program long enough?" By the end of the meeting, I was feeling like a pincushion.

"Well, there's good news and bad news about what you're proposing," Thomas Kottke told me afterward. Kottke was a nationally recognized expert in population health. "The bad news is that you don't belong to the scientific establishment and you don't really know what you're doing. But the good news is that this very fact may be the reason that your project succeeds."

His point was that every attempt to change the long-term health habits of American communities during the past few decades had failed, including the Minnesota Heart Health Program. Maybe it was time to try something new.

A TOWN IN SEARCH OF AN IDENTITY

With its tree-lined streets, seven beautiful lakes, and quaint downtown district, Albert Lea looked like a picture-postcard Midwestern town. On a typical summer weekend a handful of bikers and joggers circled the five-mile loop around the lakes, while families enjoyed boating, fishing, or waterskiing. During the first week in August the Freeborn County Fair drew more than 90,000 people to town with old-fashioned tractor pulls, livestock exhibits, crafts displays, and a carnival for the kids. "The town is big enough that you don't know everybody at the grocery store," said Tim Engstrom, who edits the *Albert Lea Tribune*. "But it's small enough that you can go into the editor's office at the newspaper and talk his ear off for half an hour."

But things were different here only a few decades ago. Back then Albert Lea was known as a meatpacking town. Since the beginning of the 20th century, the largest employer in town had been a packing plant, where cattle, hogs, and sheep were slaughtered, cut up, and packaged.

"This was a very blue-collar town," said Dennis Dieser, executive director at the Albert Lea Family YMCA. During the 1960s and 1970s, the biggest plant employed more than 1,600 people. Generations of townspeople had worked there. The jobs paid well, but they wore people out. "The workers were all under union contracts," Dieser said. "Good or bad, there was a very strong union mentality at that time." If you were a manager, you didn't talk to workers and vice versa.

Albert Lea had been founded as a commercial center for farmers, processing crops and providing seeds. The town got its name from Albert Miller Lea, a topographer who surveyed this part of the state in 1835 during an infantry expedition. Later, as the meat industry's fortunes rose and fell, the packing plant changed hands several times, and its workforce gradually shrank. Then on July 8, 2001, an event took place that cast a shadow over Albert Lea—one that residents were still struggling to emerge from. The plant burned down.

"Sixteen fire departments from across the region responded," the newspaper reported the next morning. More than 700 people were immediately out of work. The blaze also left a void in Albert Lea's spirit and identity. The town of Austin, 22 miles to the east, still had the Hormel Foods headquarters. Owatonna, 35 miles to the north, had Federated Insurance. Rochester, 64 miles to the northeast, had the Mayo Clinic. But Albert Lea was no longer a packinghouse town.

To some residents, this wasn't all bad. The air smelled better, for one thing. Small and mid-size industries continued to grow, like Lou-Rich, a homegrown manufacturer of metal products, and Mrs. Gerry's Kitchen, which started out four decades before selling potato salad and coleslaw and had quietly grown into a 121,500-square-foot factory on the edge of town. Still, the change had been hard for some, and the lack of town identity made it even harder for newcomers—such as the growing number of immigrants from places like Burma and South Sudan—to become part of the community.

"Even though Albert Lea was still a small town, people didn't necessarily know each other," said Graham, the former town planner. "We said hello to our neighbors, but we didn't know them very well." That's why he spoke up at the first Blue Zones meeting, he said. He knew that Albert Lea needed to do something to pull people back together, before it was too late.

"I was afraid the town was coming apart," he said.

PHASE ONE: A FOOD MAKEOVER

At the same time that I was consulting with the experts at the University of Minnesota I was also talking with Nancy Perry Graham (no relation to Albert Lea's Bob Graham), editor of AARP's magazine in Washington, D.C. She told me that she too was interested in a community makeover, and she paved the way for a partnership with AARP and the United Health Foundation, a nonprofit dedicated to improving health and health care, which offered us $750,000 in support of our project. I enlisted Joel Spoonheim, a former city planner who had run for secretary of state of Minnesota in 2006, to help organize our team. We all got together to look at our choices for what we were calling the AARP/Blue Zones Vitality Project, and we selected Albert Lea.

In early January 2009, shortly after announcing our selection, we signed up two of the nation's top experts on eating and nutrition to be our co-directors: Brian Wansink from Cornell University's Food and Brand Lab, who for nearly two decades had studied the psychology of eating, and Leslie Lytle, a dietary expert from the University of Minnesota. We wanted to give the town a smart food makeover.

A forest of fast-food restaurants lined the streets of Albert Lea. Other restaurants offered plate-size pancakes, meat-packed pizzas, and chicken-fried steaks covered with creamy country gravy—all foods guaranteed to pack on the pounds. Our research had shown that communities with strong leadership and dedicated citizens could proactively reduce their obesity rates. We wanted Albert Lea's population of 18,500 to emulate the healthiest towns in America, where these rates were only 17.6 percent, rather than the worst, where they were as high as 38.5 percent. Wansink's research had shown that few people grasp the real reasons they consume what they do. "Everyone—every single one of us—eats how much we eat largely because of what's around us," he wrote in his book *Mindless Eating: Why We Eat More Than We Think.* "We overeat not because of hunger but because of family and friends, packages and plates, names and numbers, labels and lights, colors and candles, shapes and smells, distractions and distances, cupboards and containers."

The upside of the way our brains work, Wansink argued, was that we could nudge ourselves into eating healthy foods just as easily as marketers do to get us to indulge in their products. "When it comes to restaurants or grocery stores, or where your kid eats, or where you work, there are a lot of small things we can do to help people eat a lot better," he said.

To spread the word in Albert Lea, Wansink visited several eateries and held a series of seminars for restaurant owners and managers. He showed them a variety of win-win solutions to reduce their operating costs and help customers be healthier. His book *Slim by Design* lists more than 100 things restaurants can do, profitably, to help people eat less. In Albert Lea we focused on just 14, and we asked the restaurants to choose 3. Restaurants could offer healthy sides such as vegetables, fruits, or salads as a default with entrées, for example, offering fries or chips only upon request. They could promote half-size portions of top-selling entrées. They could leave a pitcher of water on the table for customers just arriving, he suggested. They could serve bread before meals only if requested. They could add fresh fruit as a dessert option.

Within a few months, 30 or so food establishments had signed up with our campaign. One was the Iron Skillet at the Trails Travel Center. "We started offering fruit or salad as a side dish instead of french fries," said Cathy Purdie, director of marketing and strategic development at the Iron Skillet. When her company later did the numbers, they found that french fries orders had fallen, while sales of side salads, fruits, and vegetables had risen to take their place. The restaurant was also trying out a smaller-portion option for favorites like the three-egg omelet, she said. "Not that hungry?" the new menu asked. "Enjoy a two-egg omelet." Customers seemed to like the change.

A New, Improved Local Grocery

When the Blue Zones Project came to town, Amy Pleimling knew she needed to get involved. As the community dietician at the local Hy-Vee grocery store, she had firsthand knowledge of the town's eating habits. "It seemed like, with most people, there was a huge disconnect when it came to nutrition," she said. "They knew what to do, but they weren't actually doing it. Some were walking around a hundred pounds overweight and not even exercising."

Working with Leslie Lytle from the University of Minnesota, she began thinking of ways to make healthy foods easier to find at the Hy-Vee. Her store manager was on board, telling her to "go for it." She began by identifying "longevity foods"—products such as beans, sunflower seeds, and green tea—and tagging them with labels that stuck out from the shelves. "We call those shelf talkers," Pleimling said. Then she started holding cooking classes once a month to show residents how to include more fish, fruits, and vegetables in their diets. As customers entered the store, she made sure they were offered shopping lists of healthy foods, organized by their location in the store.

It turned out to be a good business decision. Monthly sales figures for some 30 items tagged with longevity labels later showed an average increase of 46 percent compared to the previous year. Customers could choose a specially designated Blue Zones checkout lane with display racks offering only healthy foods such as nuts, sweet potato chips, hummus, applesauce, diced peaches, and dried fruit rather than chewing gum, candy, and trashy magazines. This caused a bump in sales too.

"Plus, we got a lot of great comments," Pleimling said. Good sales, good health, and good community spirit.

"It's just neat to see," Purdie said. "It makes you wonder if the options just needed to be presented to the public—just to make it easy for them."

At the same time that Wansink was coaching restaurants, Lytle, our other co-director, was meeting with school administrators to lobby for healthier food choices in schools. Decades of research by the Coordinated Approach to Childhood Health (CATCH) Program had shown that physical activity, nutrition education, and healthy food choices could prevent childhood obesity.

One of the most important things schools can do to improve student health is to make sure kids don't have food or beverages in the hallways, Lytle told them. Schools should also prohibit food or beverages in the classrooms, and they should quit using foods as incentives or rewards. That goes for fund-raisers too: Selling candy to raise money is sending the wrong message.

We later learned that, following Lytle's advice, three of the town's elementary schools had replaced fund-raisers involving candy sales with "walking marathons" in which kids got donations for participating. One school raised $20,000—every penny of which it got to keep.

THE BIG KICKOFF

As the food makeover continued, our team was putting the rest of our strategy into action: lobbying for changes in public policies and working on ways to nudge people into moving daily, socializing more, connecting more with others, and reconnecting with their spiritual sides. Spoonheim was meeting regularly with committees of volunteers, who were doing most of the groundwork. There was a committee on schools, another on restaurants and grocery stores, a third on businesses and work sites, and a fourth on city policies.

"We knew early on that we weren't going to change the community from the outside," Spoonheim said. "The community was going to have to change itself." So besides the activists on our committees, we set out to enlist—as Puska had done in North Karelia—"ambassadors," residents who were passionate about Albert Lea and what we were trying to achieve. Our goal was to sign up 50 ambassadors, but at our first orientation meeting nearly 100 showed up. Eventually we had to cut the number off at 150.

A lot of our energy at this point was going into planning a big kickoff event in May 2009. Until now, our team had been working largely behind the scenes. But at the kickoff we wanted to introduce the Blue Zones concept to the community at large. We were hoping that at least 500 people would turn out. Instead, 1,300 people crowded into the theater. "I don't think I've ever seen a gathering of any sort here, before or since, as large as that Blue Zones gathering at the high school," said newspaper editor Engstrom.

Our speakers were a huge hit. Wansink talked about successful food makeovers. Dan Burden, a leading expert at making communities walkable and bikeable, talked about those possibilities in Albert Lea. (For more on how Burden works, see chapter 9, pages 139–143.) Nancy Graham from AARP was there, as was author and executive coach Richard Leider and his colleague, Barbara Hoese, who were planning a series of "purpose workshops" (see chapter 8, pages 124–127) in Albert Lea.

After all these inspirational speakers came my turn to take the stage. My job was to introduce the personal pledge. "You've seen what the Blue Zones is all about," I told them. "We've told you how it works. Now I'm going to ask you to take a pledge." I told them there was a form in their starter bag to enroll in the project at no cost. All they had to do was to promise to try at least 4 of the 14 activities we listed to improve their health and happiness. Among our suggestions: Take our shopping list to the grocery store to buy plant-based foods; switch to smaller bowls and dinner plates at home; turn off the television during meals; grow a garden; volunteer. I didn't tell them that evening, but every one of our ideas was based on evidence-based research. We knew that if people stuck with these simple nudges, they'd begin forming long-term healthy habits.

"We're going to take a short break now," I told them. "If you think this project is right for you, then come back. If not, you can slip out. There's no judgment."

Almost all of them came back. I asked them to stand up and look at their neighbors. "Go ahead, say hello, make eye contact," I said. I knew from research that this sort of connection creates a commitment of sorts. "You're in now. You're part of the solution."

Applause erupted. When they sat down, I introduced them to the checklists that gave them evidence-based ways to rearrange their kitchens, bedrooms, yards, and even social lives in semipermanent ways to favor good health (see chapter 12, pages 205–227). I also told them about the Vitality Compass, our online tool to assess their health and longevity, which asked them to answer 36 questions about their habits and lifestyle. We'd developed the tool with researchers at the University of Minnesota, who had based each question on the latest scientific findings and formulated the algorithms that calculated a person's life span. (The Blue Zones Vitality Compass is free and available to anyone online at *apps.bluezones.com/vitality.*)

Finally, as the crowd filed out of the auditorium and gym, we invited everyone to stop by our booths to sign up for a host of activities, from community gardens to cooking classes—and something we called "walking *moais.*"

PHASE TWO: CIRCLES OF FRIENDS

I had observed the lifelong effects of a moai while visiting Gozei Shinzato and others in Okinawa. There, a moai is a group of lifelong friends who help each other through thick and thin. Historically, moais began as a way for villagers to support one another financially, but their meaning had evolved. The centenarians I met there had built incredible social networks thanks to the tradition. I will always remember the afternoon I spent with five women who had gotten together almost daily to have tea, gossip, and share advice since they were little girls. "It's much easier to go through life knowing there is a safety net," one had told me.

But would the moai concept work in Middle America? Shortly after the kickoff event, we held rallies at four schools to invite residents to create their own walking moais, small groups that would get together on a regular basis. AARP already had a popular walking program in place, but these moais were not just about walking. They were about forging long-term relationships. We tried to match up people with similar interests and encouraged them to walk, talk, support one another, and do things such as volunteering together.

This piece of the Blue Zones plan was founded on evidence-based research as well. James Prochaska, a professor of psychology at the University of Rhode Island, had shown that, when it comes to changing health behavior, people go through stages of readiness. Some are unwilling to get up from the TV no matter what, others will run marathons without prompting, and everyone else is somewhere in between. For our moais, we assumed that the people who showed up for the program were ready to make a change in their health habits.

We also knew from work by Nicholas A. Christakis and James M. Fowler that health behaviors may be contagious. If you hang out with overweight people, you may be more likely to be heavy yourself. If you hang out with smokers, you're more likely to keep smoking. The reverse is true too. So we wanted to help people in Albert Lea curate their social networks, to interact with more people like them who wanted to be healthy and happy.

Before long, more than 800 individuals were taking part in small walking moais. Not only were they building hundreds of new friendships—often between people who otherwise might never have crossed paths—but they were also contributing to the well-being of Albert Lea by generating more than 2,200 hours of community service. As the moais become part of the fabric of the Albert Lea community, they inspired potluck meals as well. Walking, contributing, eating together: It all happened organically as part of community change.

At about the same time, we launched another social engagement initiative, the "walking school bus" program to nudge the community, young and old, into walking and socializing more. The idea behind a walking school bus was simply that a group of children would walk together to school, accompanied by parents, grandparents, teachers, or other adults. In Albert Lea, parents and teachers formed walking school buses at several elementary schools, with the goal of getting 30 percent of the kids in town walking to school.

The Power of Choice

"The Blue Zones Project made sense to me. It spoke to my heart," said Chris Chalmers, director of community education in Albert Lea. "Take food, for example. We were already eating a pretty healthy diet at our house. But now, as much as possible, our food is organic, local, raw, and fresh. We don't have pop at our house any more. Sure, we might have a frozen pizza once in a while, but it's the exception and not the rule."

As one of the original community organizers of the Blue Zones Project in Albert Lea, Chalmers said that it was the flexibility of the initiative that most impressed him. "It wasn't *you have to give up meat,* or you have to do this or that. It was a menu that allowed people to choose, what do you want to work on?" he said. "That's why I think the project can be successful across the United States. Every community can be a little bit different. It can go to a meatpacking place like Albert Lea or it can go to a vegetarian community and be successful."

Chalmers and his wife, Jennifer, have three school-age sons. "What the Blue Zones Project did for my family was to change our mind-set," he said. "My kids had never walked to school. We had never biked to church. That was two miles to church, a mile and a half to school. But the Blue Zones was sort of a trigger. We started biking to church. The kids started walking to school, not every day with the walking school bus group, but with one friend or two friends.

"The bottom line is we don't have to live in Okinawa or Greece to be healthy," he said. "We can take these concepts and implement them in our community. I want this to be a great place for my kids to grow up in and for our family and friends to live in."

At Lakeview Elementary School, for example, two different groups created walking school buses, which they named the Lakeview Locomotive and the Park Avenue Express. "It was a sight to see—a trail of almost 40 children on a rainy Wednesday walking with their parents and teachers," the *Albert Lea Tribune* reported on May 14, 2009. "Some wore ponchos and others carried umbrellas, as they walked from Hatch Bridge, around Fountain Lake, past Monkey Island and eventually to the school."

Besides boosting the health of Albert Lea's youngest citizens, the walking school bus program also created opportunities for some of its oldest ones. With parents and teachers so busy these days, we tapped the community's senior population to serve as chaperones for students as they walked to school. Everyone got more exercise, and the older folks discovered a new sense of purpose. As research by Linda P. Fried, dean of Columbia University's Mailman School of Public Health, has shown, seniors who volunteer are not only doing good for their communities, they may also be improving their own mental and physical health. "Giving back to your community may slow the aging process in ways that lead to a higher quality of life in older adults," Fried has said.

It was another win-win situation for Blue Zones Project participants in Albert Lea.

IT'S A WRAP

"Good morning to you from Albert Lea," Kate Snow said to the TV camera on a chilly October morning. The weekend co-anchor of ABC's *Good Morning America (GMA)* was standing in the gazebo at Fountain Lake, surrounded by a cheerful group of onlookers, including several of our project's most active volunteers—and yours truly. It was the second time in three months that *GMA* had broadcast live from Albert Lea, which had raised everybody's spirits. In July Sam Champion had given the national weather forecast from the Brookside Education Center, where 500 or so residents, most wearing bright blue T-shirts, had joined him at dawn. People here were getting the message that their health makeover experiment mattered to the rest of the country.

Our ten months in Albert Lea were drawing to a close—even though many of the initiatives we'd launched would be continued for years by members of the community.

"You did even better than you expected," Snow said to me as the TV camera broadcast our image across the nation. Roughly 800 people had used the Vitality Compass both before and after the project, giving us a chance to estimate changes in life expectancy. "You were hoping to add two years onto people's lives and you have added . . ."

"Three point one years," I said, finishing her sentence.

Not only that, participants had also reported losing an average of 2.8 pounds. They told us they were eating more vegetables and seafood and experiencing fewer days of depression. The town had made big gains in smoking policies too: Before the project, only 4 percent of employees in Albert Lea worked on tobacco-free grounds; now that number was 24 percent, and by early 2014 it would reach 40 percent. Absenteeism was down by 20 percent at some businesses, and officials had reported a big drop in city workers' health care costs. New bike paths were planned on city streets and around the lakes.

"This has been a huge movement," said Randy Kehr, executive director of the Albert Lea Chamber of Commerce. "It has reconnected our community in a way that I never thought possible."

These were rough indicators, to be sure. I wish we could have taken everybody's blood pressure and measured their cholesterol levels, as Kane had recommended. I wish we could have brought in a firm like Gallup to apply their advanced metrics tools, as we've done in communities since Albert Lea. But they were still outstanding numbers—far better than we had expected—and all pointing in the right direction. It was as if a kid who'd worked hard and was afraid he'd get a C had ended up with an A instead.

"It was amazing. All these changes were coming right from the community in a real, organic way," Lytle said. "This project showed me that as researchers we can be part of change instead of just pointing to the direction of change."

The truly amazing thing was that nothing we did in Albert Lea was huge. Nothing took a ton of effort. It was the sum of little changes that moved the dial so dramatically.

At the wrap-up event at the high school, I asked people to stand up if they felt healthier, and a lot of them did. I asked them if they'd made changes in their houses. I asked them if they were eating healthier foods. More people stood. Then I asked them to stand up if they'd made a new friend. About 95 percent of the auditorium stood up—which gave me the chills.

You know why?

Because when it comes to longevity, there's no quick fix—and friends last.

MEASURES OF SUCCESS IN ALBERT LEA, MINNESOTA

The night before Kate Snow's TV broadcast from the Fountain Lake gazebo in Albert Lea, we announced the results of our efforts to the public. We were not disappointed.

- About 4,000 people—roughly a fourth of all adults in Albert Lea—had signed the Blue Zones pledge, taken the Vitality Compass, or participated in one of our activities.
- More than half of all employers in town were acting on pledges to make their workplaces healthier environments, affecting more than 4,300 employees.
- About 1,400 children—100 percent of the students in grades three through eight—had been reached through at least one of our Blue Zones school programs.
- At least 800 people had joined some 70 walking moais, logging an estimated 37,558 miles together.
- More than two-thirds of Albert Lea's 34 locally owned or operated restaurants were making changes to help patrons eat healthier.
- Community gardens blossomed from 70 to 116.
- More than 80 children, attending five different schools, went to school and home again as part of a walking school bus.

CHAPTER EIGHT

❧

Thriving in the Beach Cities

LAUNCHING A BLUE ZONES PROJECT in the Los Angeles area posed big challenges for us, the first of which was its geography. The South Bay region is a jumble of industry and beaches. Just south of the runways at LAX, past the massive storage tanks of Chevron's El Segundo Refinery, are some of the most appealing and coveted stretches of oceanfront real estate in the nation. The result: a congested pressure cooker of stress.

Three towns here, each with the word "beach" in their name, invited us to join them in a community-wide health experiment. Bordering the Pacific on one side and freeways on the other, these Beach Cities, as they were called—Manhattan Beach, Hermosa Beach, and Redondo Beach— had much in common. All three were once home to simple cottages and surf shops but were now filled with pricey houses and brokerage offices. Manhattan Beach, closest to downtown L.A., was the most expensive. In mid-2014, the average listing price for a home was just under $3 million.

"Real estate is a religion here," said Mark McDermott, editor of the *Easy Reader,* which covers the South Bay region. "Even if people aren't in the real estate market, they follow the listings for sport." An easygoing native Iowan with a blond ponytail and beard, McDermott reported on all aspects of life in the Beach Cities. This morning he was pedaling an old beach cruiser bike the wrong way down a one-way backstreet in

Manhattan Beach. As he coasted down the hill, he offered an insider's perspective on the three communities.

Although a lot alike, these towns had many differences too, McDermott pointed out. "Each of the Beach Cities has a pier, and the pier reflects the personality of each community," he said. The one in Manhattan Beach, for example, had a quaint gazebo at the end where residents could relax and drink their lattes. That suited the 36,000 overachievers who lived here, he said.

Hermosa Beach, by contrast, was the party town. Just to the south of Manhattan Beach, it had a minimalist pier, anchored by a plaza filled with souvenir shops and beach bars. "It used to be a bohemian place," McDermott said, with jazz clubs and hip coffee shops. With only about 20,000 residents, it was the smallest of the three towns and home to more young people: waiters, hairdressers, and aspiring actors.

Finally, Redondo Beach was the largest, with 68,000 residents. It was also the most diverse, with sizable Hispanic and Asian populations. Its pier, known as a gang hangout in the 1980s, was destroyed by a fire in 1988 and rebuilt in 1995 as a sprawling tourist attraction with shops and restaurants.

What united these three towns, of course, was the ocean. On any given morning, down by the water, people were out on the Strand—the concrete sidewalk that runs along the beach—from joggers and in-line skaters to bicyclists and dog walkers. In a place like this, with all the sunshine and fresh air, you might think that community leaders wouldn't need to encourage people to stay active and eat healthy foods. But looks can be deceiving, McDermott said.

For every person at the beach, there were dozens more battling traffic on the nearby Pacific Coast Highway or San Diego Freeway. For working families struggling to make ends meet, the beach might as well not exist. Even for wealthy professionals, with their busy schedules, getting to the beach may not be a priority. "The ones you see jogging or biking are simply the most visible ones," McDermott said. "There are many others sitting at home watching TV or eating a lot of bad food."

Despite their enviable location, in other words, the Beach Cities weren't immune to the same pressures and bad habits that afflicted the rest of the nation.

A NEW CHALLENGE

Following our success in Albert Lea, Minnesota, our Blue Zones team sent information packets to the mayors of about 300 communities across the United States, inviting them to apply for the next phase of the project. Over the course of three years, we told them, we planned to use what we'd learned in Albert Lea to transform another community. The question was, did they want in? The answer from 55 of them: a resounding yes.

None of this would have been happening if it hadn't been for Ben Leedle, Jr., CEO of Healthways, a for-profit health care company. After hearing about the Albert Lea story and reading my *Blue Zones* book, he'd reached out to us with a bold idea. Why not try the experiment again in a bigger community—to prove that it wasn't a fluke? If it worked, he said, it might become the biggest thing in health care in the next generation.

What Leedle knew from his work at Healthways was that a transformation was taking place in the nation's medical establishment. The "fee for service" model, in which doctors and hospitals were compensated for everything they did to fight diseases, was rapidly being replaced by the "accountable care" model, in which health care providers were compensated for keeping a population of patients healthy. Instead of being paid for every test and procedure they ordered, physicians and hospitals more and more were being rewarded for producing good outcomes.

To make this new approach work financially, every effort had to be made to reduce the number of patients getting sick. That's where Albert Lea came in. We'd demonstrated that, with the right mix of policies and programs, we could help improve the health of an entire community. As far as we knew, the Blue Zones team was the only one who'd ever done that. Leedle was impressed enough by our success to make us an offer: If we were willing to spend the next few years applying what we'd learned from those results to transform one or more communities, and doing it in a way that could be measured and confirmed scientifically, then Healthways would support us financially. It was an offer we couldn't refuse.

By late summer 2010 we'd winnowed the 55 candidate cities down to a handful. We knew that our chances for success would be greatest if we picked a city eager for change. So we visited each of the finalist cities several times, talking with civic leaders at all levels. In the end, the Beach Cities stood out as the perfect choice, not only because the population there was active and well educated, but also because the community was served by an organization called the Beach Cities Health District (BCHD), whose goals seemed to be perfectly aligned with our own.

The BCHD had a unique history. Created in 1955, its original purpose was to build and operate a hospital for South Bay residents at a time when medical facilities were scarce in this part of L.A. County. That purpose changed in 1998, when competition forced the hospital to close. The good news for residents was that the BCHD had a sizable endowment from investments, which it could now refocus on a new mission: keeping the South Bay population *out* of hospitals. Instead of treating illnesses, the BCHD dedicated itself to keeping people healthy.

In September we officially announced the Beach Cities as our choice. The BCHD board would be our sponsor, contributing $1.8 million over three years, while Healthways agreed to provide $3.5 million. It was time to roll up our sleeves and get to work. The first order of business was to establish a health baseline to measure our progress. We asked our colleagues at the Gallup company to do a series of surveys, using a tool they'd developed with Healthways called the Well-Being Index. Since the index was launched in 2008, Gallup had used it to measure the health and happiness of more than two million American adults. California currently ranked 18th. Through phone interviews with 1,200 randomly selected residents in the Beach Cities per year from 2010 through 2013, the index measured six categories:

- Life Evaluation
- Emotional Health
- Physical Health
- Healthy Behaviors
- Work Environment
- Basic Access (meaning access to health care, money for necessities, and so on)

Averaging these domains produced an overall well-being score.

When the Gallup survey numbers for the Beach Cities came in, they turned up a few surprises. Although residents here compared favorably with averages for California or the United States, there was room for improvement in a few key areas, such as body weight and emotional health. Sixty percent of Beach Cities residents reported being over-weight—not much better than the national average of 66 percent. More alarming, when asked if they were feeling stress, anger, or worries in their lives, about half of those polled said yes. In fact, of 188 communities studied by Gallup, the Beach Cities ranked near the bottom for self-reported anger and worrying. The numbers were so bad, Gallup reported, it suggested that Beach Cities residents were angrier than people in Detroit and as worried as those in post-Katrina New Orleans.

"I wasn't surprised that our stress numbers were higher than normal," said Lisa Santora, chief medical officer of the BCHD. "But some of the highest in the country? I would never have expected that."

To others in the Beach Cities, the "stressed out" label came as no shock. "We live in this beautiful place, but we're all on edge," said Jeff Duclos, former mayor of Hermosa Beach. He mainly blamed traffic. "We're stuck in the middle of this huge metropolis, Los Angeles, which is completely dysfunctional in terms of moving people around." For nearly two decades Duclos had commuted 30 to 40 miles between the Beach Cities and places like West L.A., where he worked in the enter-tainment industry. Fighting the traffic every morning and evening had been "completely debilitating," he said. He'd arrive at work angry and get home exhausted.

Then one day he had enough, he said. He decided to run his consult-ing business from his home in Hermosa Beach and teach at UCLA and California State University, Northridge. So now, instead of doing battle on the freeways each morning, he got a dog and started taking it for long walks. "It profoundly changed my life in a positive way," he said. The Gallup numbers were a wake-up call, he added. "We really weren't who we thought we were in the Beach Cities. The Blue Zones was going to give us a way to become the community we wanted to be."

FOOD, BIKES, AND PURPOSE

Aiming to repeat the success we had in Albert Lea, we turned once more to our brain trust of experts to energize local residents. We started again with food, bringing back Brian Wansink of Cornell's Food and Brand Lab, a co-director of the Blue Zones Project, to meet with restaurant owners and managers.

One of those owners was Alex Jordan of Eat at Joe's, a popular diner in Redondo Beach. Known for its big portions, Eat at Joe's was the home of the "John Wayne" breakfast special, which consisted of two eggs, sausages, and cheese smothered in Spanish sauce on top of a bed of home fries. After listening to Wansink's suggestions about how to make more money with healthier options, Jordan decided to offer half-size portions of many dishes, as well as making fruits and salads side dishes instead of fries. "We had a healthier section in our menu before, but now we've kind of expanded it and made it more promi-nent," Jordan told the *Easy Reader*. "We try to make it easier to make healthier choices, like ground turkey instead of ground beef, or egg whites instead of eggs. People seem to like it, and it has made money, so it covers all the bases."

To talk about the physical layout of the Beach Cities, we also asked Dan Burden to take residents on walking tours to show them how to make their streets more walkable and bike friendly (read more on Burden's work in chapter 9, pages 139–143). And, finally, we brought in Richard Leider to hold "purpose workshops," where residents could take stock of their gifts and aspirations to increase their satisfaction with life.

Considering the size of the stress problem in the Beach Cities, Leider was exactly what these towns needed. As I'd discovered during my visits to the world's Blue Zones, a sense of purpose was essential to achieving a long, healthy life. *Ikigai* in Okinawa, *plan de vida* in Costa Rica—so many of the centenarians I had met in the world's Blue Zones were aware of the importance of their own "reason for living," as the Okinawan word translates. And in the United States, nobody understood the power of purpose better than Richard Leider. In fact, I've often referred to him

Rethinking the Menu

When Richard Crespin heard about the Blue Zones Project, he thought it sounded like trouble. As chef at Baleen Kitchen in the Portofino Hotel & Marina in Redondo Beach, he didn't take kindly to suggestions about what to put on his menu. He knew that the last thing most customers chose from a menu was something boring labeled "healthy." But the directive had come straight from the Portofino's general manager, who wanted the hotel to become part of the Blue Zones effort.

Crespin suggested they add to the menu a simple plate of raw vegetables—sliced carrots, zucchini, green peppers. Nobody was excited.

"Then I thought, if I'm going to do this, I need to come up with something that will really stand out," Crespin said. "So I kind of went back to my roots." He remembered how his grandmother used to cook vegetables when he was growing up in San Sebastián, Spain. Everything was fresh. Everything was seasonal. In many ways, he thought, the traditional methods were also the healthiest ones. "I started looking at mushrooms and brussels sprouts to see if they could stand on their own as an entrée. Maybe I'd make a napoleon out of mushrooms. They give you a feeling in your mouth that tricks your mind into thinking you're eating a heartier protein. Or beets, or carrots, or cauliflower. When you roast a cauliflower, it takes on so many different nuances."

The Blue Zones challenge also prompted him to reconsider the rest of his menu. "How can I make my chicken crispy, but lighten the load on cholesterol and fats?" he wondered. His solution: Brown the chicken in a frying pan without any oil or butter, then finish cooking it in the oven. "Or what if I used a vegetable puree to thicken a sauce instead of throwing butter or cream on it?" If the community was asking for a healthier option, he would find a way to give it to them. And the best way to do that would be to keep it low-key.

"I wasn't standing on a soapbox saying, This is a better way to eat," he said. "I was just saying, Try this. And people liked it. So I said, Great, try it again."

as the Pope of Purpose. His message: Clarify your purpose and you reduce your stress.

It was standing room only the night of his first workshop at the Redondo Beach Performing Arts Center, which had a capacity of 1,500 people. "Purpose is fundamental to health, healing, longevity, and happiness," Leider told the crowd. "But often it can be hard to get your hands around. I have specific tools and practices to help you do that."

Leider introduced the group to a 15-minute exercise he called Calling Cards, which he said would help them understand their gifts, passions, and values. He passed out decks of cards, each of which had a phrase on it describing a talent or gift. Here are some examples:

- Seeing the big picture
- Getting to the heart of matters
- Creating things
- Analyzing information
- Awakening spirit
- Instructing people
- Creating trust
- Breaking molds
- Making deals
- Bringing out potential

"Spread the cards in front of you," he told the group. "Then sort them into three piles: yes, maybe, and no. Finally, choose the top five that describes your gift or passion best."

After they'd done that, he asked each person to discuss his or her number one choice with another person in the crowd—to describe how they applied their gift or talent to accomplish things they cared about. "All of a sudden the energy in the room went up," Leider said. "The whole room lit up." People were curious about each other's choices. What are your top five gifts? What are my top five? How well do we really know each other? "When they put it into their own words and applied it to their own experiences, they started to see their natural passions," Leider said. "They started to see purpose as a real, living, breathing thing rather than as a concept or something philosophical or spiritual. They saw it as something very practical."

"What if you could harness the energy in this room?" Leider asked the group. What would it be like to live in a community where, instead of dreading traffic or going to work, people were fully engaged with their gifts, passions, and values? "Knowing why we get up in the morning is one of the great antidotes to the downs in life," he said.

MAKING A DIFFERENCE

At the same time that Leider was coaching residents to sharpen their sense of purpose, the rest of our Blue Zones team was working with policymakers, business owners, school officials, and many others to reshape other key aspects of life in the Beach Cities.

As a result of our lobbying, the Hermosa Beach City Council passed an ordinance banning smoking at beaches or other outdoor areas, including the city pier, public parks, dining areas, and parking lots. The Manhattan Beach City Council likewise passed a policy forbidding smoking in public places citywide. The Redondo Beach City Council approved a dramatic expansion of bike paths. Restaurants created healthier menus. Children were walking to school every day, and people were making new friends and getting together to eat, walk, and work together as volunteers.

As a show of their support, the mayors of the three Beach Cities competed against one another in a cook-off at Abigaile, a local restaurant. The contest was modeled after the *Iron Chef* TV show, with each mayor teaming up with a community chef and preparing a vegetarian dish in 30 minutes or less, using a secret ingredient that wasn't revealed to them until just before the contest began. (It turned out to be green lentils.) Wayne Powell, mayor of Manhattan Beach, and Chris Garasic, chef of Zinc restaurant, won first prize with jicama enchiladas that were stuffed with coconut and raw almond cheese and served over a lentil puree and topped off with cilantro pesto and tropical slaw. The crowd also cheered the runners-up—ravioli filled with a Mediterranean blend of lentils, feta, olives, and raisins, and sautéed oyster mushrooms with lentil tabbouleh and avocado chocolate mousse.

Would any of these things have happened if we hadn't brought the Blue Zones Project to the Beach Cities? Most people already knew that smoking was bad, walking was good, and fast food was convenient but not helpful for your waistline. But we'd nudged these communities into recognizing that residents could tackle these issues in new ways, and the impacts of our efforts were radiating through these towns like ripples in a pond.

Consider what was happening at Hermosa View School, where principal Silvia Gluck had instituted several new initiatives, from walking school buses to student gardens to lessons in mindfulness. Gluck had 483 students in three grades at her school: kindergarten, first, and second. As she left her office one morning, she waded through a crowd of students carrying their lunches to picnic tables outside. This was California, after all, where they do everything in the sunshine. Gluck glanced at their paper plates to see what students had taken from the salad bar in the breezeway.

"Look at all that corn. Way to go!" she said to one girl. "Good for you," she said to another. "You took a banana!"

When a boy passed by with a plate piled high with chicken fingers from the cafeteria—and nothing from the salad bar—she stopped him with a gentle hand on his shoulder. "Where's your fruit or vegetable?" she asked.

"I dropped it," he said unconvincingly.

"Well, go back and find something else," she suggested.

Making fruits and vegetables an easy lunch option was only one of the many changes Gluck had welcomed to Hermosa View. Another was the MindUP program, an initiative sponsored by the Hawn Foundation and the actress Goldie Hawn to promote academic success through emotional awareness and regulation. Besides teaching kids about the biological functions of the brain, the program also coached students on ways to control their emotions and develop empathy for others. "If a child doesn't feel safe, optimistic, hopeful . . . they're not going to learn," Goldie Hawn, actress and founder of the program, told one interviewer.

The Doctor

Before coming to the Beach Cities Health District, where she was chief medical officer, Santora had worked as a physician at a neighborhood clinic in nearby Venice, California. In her role there, she'd felt frustrated by her limited success at helping patients improve their diets. "As a physician I had all these tools to encourage patients to eat better," she said. "But the minute they left my office, they faced a cart selling *chich-arrones*—fried pig skins—right outside the family clinic." You could see it at any hospital too, she said. "I'd be treating a patient for a stroke and their family would be eating food full of trans fats and all of these other horrible things right in the hospital cafeteria."

As much as her patients might have wanted to adopt a healthier lifestyle, in other words, everything all around them was pushing them in another direction, down the wrong road. "I realized that many of the changes we needed to be making were out in the community," she said. But the health care system wasn't very good yet at addressing the big picture. That's why the Blue Zones Project was so valuable. It shifted the focus to the environment, to making it easier to obtain healthy foods and to stay active. "As a health care professional, I find that there are a lot of public domain resources out there—pamphlets on nutrition and diet plans. But there's something aspirational about the Blue Zones Project," she said. "People want to be a part of it."

"There's a lot of stress on children these days, because we're in a very stressful environment," Gluck said. "But are we teaching students when or how to decompress?" Since MindUP was introduced at Hermosa View three years ago, Gluck had seen impressive results, she said. Now, whenever there was some kind of problem between students that required the attention of the principal, she took a mindful approach.

"I never ask, 'What did you do?'" she explained. "That's not the right way to approach a child. I usually ask, 'Were you mindful in your decision-making? Were you mindful in your conversation?' And they always think about it. Sometimes they'll say, 'My prefrontal cortex wasn't working.' This is coming out of a first grader's mouth or a kindergartener! And I'll ask, 'Well, why wasn't it working?' Then I'll say, 'Give me an example of how we can fix this.'"

Besides reducing the stress levels in class and on the playground, she said, MindUP had another beneficial impact: "I don't have as many kids in my office."

BACK TO BASICS

As our project continued to reach more deeply into these communities, residents were figuring out their own ways to avoid the high-pressure rat race. Take Nancy Fulton Rogers, for example. For more than 20 years, the Hermosa Beach resident thrived on a steady diet of stress. As a freelance producer of TV commercials, she worked 12 to 14 hours a day, commuting to Hollywood. When she wasn't fighting traffic on the freeways, she was multitasking on airplanes, winging toward some distant location for a shoot. "It was impossible to have a balanced life in my business," she said. "You had to be full on. There was no time for a healthy diet or socializing. Everything else suffered."

When the economy tanked a few years ago, her phone stopped ringing. Jobs dried up. She thought, What do I do now? Although she and her husband had lived in Hermosa Beach for almost 18 years, she didn't have close friends there. It hadn't been a priority for her when she'd been so busy. Then she heard about the Blue Zones walking *moais*.

"It piqued my interest," she said, "especially the idea of meeting other people in my community. Having a tribe was something I was missing."

Fulton Rogers went to an organizational meeting at Mira Costa High School in Manhattan Beach, where she met the half dozen other women who were also interested in walking. They decided to meet once a week at the Hermosa Beach Community Center and walk for an hour or so. "Pretty soon we were like glue," she said. "We'd walk in pairs and just gab about stuff. We'd talk about our animals. Our grandchildren. Our houses. We were all relatively fit and we kept up a fast pace. We were on a mission."

About the same time, Fulton Rogers decided to enroll in cooking school. If it worked out, she was considering becoming a private chef or caterer. So she invited her walking moai to become her guinea pigs and held a cooking class for them. She taught them how to make four or five Blue Zones–worthy dishes—everything plant based. Her passion rippled through the community, influencing the eating choices of her moai, and then reaching those women's families and friends. "They loved it," she said. "And so did I."

When Leider came to town, Fulton Rogers and several members of her moai went to a purpose workshop together. "For us it was like digging in a little deeper and finding out even more about each other," she said. "We opened up a little more. After one of us shared something very personal, the rest of us felt like we could too."

Eventually her TV work revived and her phone started ringing again with jobs in Hollywood. But Fulton Rogers didn't intend to get back on the same treadmill as before. "I'm producing again, all food related. But I'm also cooking and doing other things," she said. "It's great to wear different hats. Looking back, I realize now that keeping a tribe intact is something you must keep working at. It doesn't come easy. If you want to make changes, they have to be ones you do daily or you'll slide right back into the same old ruts."

Life was still a challenge, Fulton Rogers said. But she'd always liked a good challenge. And, besides, she had a tribe now to watch her back.

A NICE BUMP

As the fall of 2013 approached and our three-year effort in the Beach Cities was nearing its conclusion, we asked the Gallup team to conduct a final community health checkup. Our sense was that we'd made a difference here. But would the numbers tell the same story?

We weren't disappointed. According to the new surveys, the Beach Cities had experienced a 14 percent drop in obesity since 2010. That represented a savings of more than $2.3 million a year in incremental health care costs, Gallup said. They'd also seen a 30 percent drop in the smoking rate (from 11 percent to 7 percent of the population), which avoided about $6.97 million a year in health care costs. The number of residents exercising regularly had risen 10 percent. Diabetes was down. High blood pressure was down. "I was really impressed," said Dan Witters, research director of the Gallup-Healthways Well-Being Index. "These communities were already doing well in many of these areas, and yet they still saw improvement."

In particular, the "life evaluation" score of the Beach Cities jumped way up, Witters said. This was the part of the survey where people were asked to rank their lives today and in the future. Their level of satisfaction with life increased about eight percentage points. By comparison, the U.S. average went up only about half of one percentage point, and the California average only a little more than one and a half percentage points during the same period. Moving the dial in the Beach Cities in this way reflected well on the Blue Zones Project's impact, Witters said. "People here think their lives are better now. That doesn't come out of thin air."

Emotional health was still a challenge in these communities. When it came to feeling stressed out and treating one another with respect, Beach Cities residents actually lost ground slightly since 2010. Clearly, there was still work to do in this area. But overall we were happy. And so was the BCHD board. Considering the impressive progress they'd seen in these communities, the BCHD board decided to continue funding the Blue Zones program on their own. "It's a rare thing when you can come up with a real measurable success like this in the public health field," Susan Burden, the CEO of BCHD, said. "We are the envy of the public health world right now."

Noel Chun, a BCHD board member, said he envisioned an even bigger potential for the Blue Zones experiment. Besides making life better for Beach Cities residents, he thought the project could eventually become a significant long-term scientific study. To change the trajectory of what's happening to the health of most Americans, you have to start somewhere, he said. "We're in a unique situation here in the Beach Cities, because of our financial stability, to become a center of excellence for preventative care and wellness. I see a very long-term commitment here."

Well, that was music to my ears. I'd always thought of the Blue Zones as a long-term experiment in social change, but it was gratifying to hear others talking about it in the same terms. We'd come a long way since my first visits to Greece, Okinawa, Sardinia, Loma Linda, and Costa Rica. With the help of so many, we'd taken the fundamental wisdom of centenarians and the research of leading scientists and created an effective program for community change right here in America. We'd done it twice now, with measurable success. But did we know enough to take what we'd learned and apply it to a broad range of other communities, some very different from wholesome Albert Lea and the affluent, well-educated Beach Cities?

We were about to find out in Iowa.

MEASURES OF SUCCESS IN THE BEACH CITIES

As part of their commitment to the Blue Zones Project, the citizens and leadership of the Beach Cities racked up a string of significant victories:

- The Redondo Beach City Council approved a plan to nearly triple the total length of bike paths, lanes, and other safe biking routes in the community from 14 to 38 miles.
- The owners and managers of more than 40 restaurants created healthy menus for their customers.
- At least 3,000 students at 13 schools began walking to class every morning, eliminating thousands of car trips a year.
- About 1,600 residents joined 150 moais and got together regularly to walk, share potluck meals, or attend purpose workshops together.

CHAPTER NINE

Blue Zoning the Pork State

T HE ANNOUNCEMENT CAME AS A SURPRISE. On August 10, 2011, Governor Terry Branstad issued a challenge to fellow Iowans to make the Hawkeye State the healthiest in the nation by 2016. At the time Iowa ranked 19th on that list. "It's an ambitious goal to jump 18 positions in 5 years," Branstad said, "but if anyone can do it, Iowans can."

Branstad, a Republican, was enormously popular. First elected in 1982, he'd been re-elected three times in a row, taken a ten-year break, then been voted back into the governor's office in 2010. "He's become like political comfort food for many of us," one Iowa newspaper columnist wrote, "sort of like mustachioed macaroni and cheese." In fact, one of the only things the governor could do to lose the affection of Iowa voters, the columnist joked, would be to mess with Iowans' access to thick steaks, bacon, buttered corn, and cold beer.

But, in fact, that wasn't too far off from what Branstad was advocating. If Iowans could make the kind of comprehensive lifestyle changes that his Healthiest State Initiative would require, the state could avoid $16 billion in health care costs over the same five-year period, he said. The new initiative wasn't going to be run by the state government, though. Just the opposite. It was going to be a grassroots effort led by communities and businesses. Branstad's role was to use the bully pulpit of his office to encourage Iowans to get involved. "Making Iowa the healthiest state in the nation is not only critical to the economic viability of our state," he said. "It is also critical to the quality of life of all Iowans."

The Blue Zones Project was a centerpiece of the effort. With up to $25 million in funding over five years of oversight and collaboration with Wellmark Blue Cross and Blue Shield, the largest insurance company in the state, the Blue Zones team and our partners at Healthways took on the task of transforming Iowa town by town. Grocery stores promoted healthy foods, restaurants redesigned menus, and workplaces upgraded vending machines—among countless other small changes—as our teams went from one community to the next making healthy choices easier through permanent changes to the environment, local policies, and social networks. In the first phase of the effort ten towns would serve as demonstration sites for the rest. Ultimately, every town and business in the state would have access to Blue Zones tools and practices.

This was a huge leap for us—making over an entire state. We'd been remarkably successful so far at transforming individual communities. But was our model scalable? Could we adapt our strategies adequately to respond to multiple towns at the same time? If not, how did we need to adjust our approach? We'd given a great deal of thought to these questions before coming to Iowa, and we'd put together what we believed to be promising solutions. But there's nothing like actually putting a plan into action to discover if it's going to work.

We began by auditioning 84 communities for the first ten slots as demonstration sites, hoping to find in each town the same combination of manageable size, committed leadership, and local resources that we'd found in Albert Lea and the Beach Cities. Then on May 4, 2012, with our partners at Wellmark and Healthways, we announced the selection of four—Spencer, Cedar Falls, Waterloo, and Mason City—as the first Blue Zones Project communities. The following January we announced six more: Muscatine, Sioux City, Cedar Rapids, Marion, Iowa City, and Oskaloosa.

Our experiences in the Beach Cities had taught us that each community was different, and we needed to account for local interpretations of the

Blue Zones model. What we were putting together, after all, wasn't so much a template for community change as it was an operating system. So as we got ready to introduce this system to Iowa communities, we got ready to encounter many new challenges too.

Compared to the relatively progressive Beach Cities, for example, we knew that Iowans were likely to be more conservative, not only in their politics but also in their attitudes toward social change. The last thing we wanted to do was to come across as a bunch of outsiders telling Iowans they needed to change. We weren't going to yank that barbecued rib from anybody's hand.

As Pekka Puska had learned in North Karelia, change had to come from the bottom up, with the Blue Zones staff engaging individuals wherever they found them, putting our "boots in the mud," as Puska called it. Our plan was to offer communities a menu of evidence-based goals they could choose from, then coach them as they pursued those goals. With respect to healthy food policies, for example, our suggestions ranged from encouraging the creation of farmers markets to promoting breastfeeding. Were there vacant lots in town? Why not turn them into community gardens? Were food trucks becoming popular at lunchtime? Maybe they should be required to include at least one healthy item on their menu, along with the usual fried foods and sugary snacks.

There was a local precedent for what we were doing—from the agricultural world. During the first years of the 20th century, a tiny beetle called the boll weevil had devastated cotton farms in the South. The pest, which was resistant to insecticides at the time, laid its eggs inside maturing cotton. Weevil larvae ate the cotton as they grew, damaging up to 90 percent of a farm's crop.

Enter Seaman Knapp, a former president of the Iowa Agricultural College (now Iowa State University) and a practitioner of hands-on education. The U.S. Department of Agriculture (USDA) enlisted him to help stem the devastating boll weevil infestation. Knapp arrived in Terrell, Texas, just east of Dallas, in 1903 and persuaded a local farmer to turn his land into a demonstration site by making a few bold changes to his farming techniques, including the use of several strains of cottonseeds.

Never Too Old

LeRoy Buehler knew he was too heavy. At six feet three inches tall, he'd always been a big man, but lately the 67-year-old Waterloo resident's weight had climbed to 400 pounds, and it was starting to worry him. Then something happened that convinced him to change his ways.

"Last summer my grandson was playing T-ball," he said. "We went to his game and the umpire didn't show up. So I said, I'll do it." But after only two innings of standing behind the plate, he had to call it quits and sit down, he said.

When they went home, he realized that his weight was threatening to cut short his life. His wife, who worked at Wellmark, told him about the Blue Zones Project coming to town. He decided to make some changes.

Buehler began by watching the portions he ate at each meal. "Initially, I didn't change what I was eating as much as I did how much I was eating," he said. "Just a smaller plate, put on it what you want, and don't go back. I quit going to the pizza places. Honest to God, I used to go in and order a large pepperoni pizza and then say to my wife, Did you want anything? Now if we go, I eat two pieces there and two pieces tomorrow at home."

By the time the Blue Zones Project officially kicked off in November 2012, Buehler had lost 50 pounds. "At that point, I hadn't even done any exercise," he said. "No walking or whatever. Initially, I couldn't have done any anyway."

Then Buehler decided to go to a walking *moai* meeting and joined a group that got together once a week at lunchtime to walk. "When we started, my friends said they used to look over their shoulder at me," Buehler said. "Now they're trying to keep up."

After a year of eating better and walking more, Buehler had lost a total of 80 pounds and had become a vocal champion of the Blue Zones way. "I'm thinking, why the heck aren't more people doing this?" he said. "Because it works. It ain't that hard."

Knapp's brilliant insight was that, if the experiment turned out to be successful, then neighboring farmers would be more likely to copy those techniques. And, of course, that's exactly what happened. While many Texas farms were going under, the demonstration farm turned a profit. Word spread, and Knapp's agricultural innovations caught on—disseminated far and wide in the coming years by extension agents trained in the new techniques.

We saw Knapp's success, and the way it propagated broadly thanks to extension agents, as a model for our own approach to community health in Iowa. If the first wave of Blue Zones towns—the ones eager and willing to change with our help—could demonstrate measurable progress in their efforts to eat better, be happier, and become more prosperous, then other towns would too.

One of the key lessons we'd learned during our community campaigns was that a town's physical design powerfully affected its quality of life. Were there enough sidewalks for residents to walk to nearby shops? Were there enough bike paths for children to pedal to school? Was it safe for pedestrians to cross busy intersections? Were public parks smoke-free? Did the town encourage community gardens and farmers markets, where fresh foods were easy to find? Whenever we first visited a community, one of the first things we did was take a close look at its "built environment"—its streets, buildings, parks and how they were all connected—to see if the town was making it easier or harder for residents to eat healthy, stay active, and generally enjoy life.

That's what Dan Burden was doing as he stretched a measuring tape across the width of a sidewalk in downtown Muscatine, Iowa, surrounded by 20 or so civic leaders. "Twelve feet," he said. "That's outstanding. I'm already in love with your town. It has great bones."

At 69, wearing hiking boots, wire rim glasses, a bushy mustache, and flyaway silver hair, Burden looked like a cross between a forest ranger and a mad scientist. During the past 16 years, as co-founder of the nonprofit Walkable and Livable Communities Institute, he'd helped more than 3,500 towns across the country become healthier and more prosperous. Since 2009 he'd been a key member of our Blue Zones team.

This morning Burden was leading a group in this small town on the Mississippi River on what he called a "walking audit." The purpose of the outing was to identify features of the 19th-century downtown—such as the width of sidewalks—that made it walkable or bikeable, as well as to suggest other ways to revitalize the area. At six feet three, wearing a neon green safety vest, Burden stood out in the crowd. As he strode down the street with his long legs, everybody hustled to keep up.

"This is a natural vista point," he said, stopping on a corner overlooking the Mississippi. "You want to keep that vista open." Muscatine is located on a bend of the river that turns sharply to the south. A century ago that gave the community a strategic advantage for loading and unloading timber, grain, and other goods. But like many river towns, Muscatine hadn't updated its waterfront recently to make the most of its potential. Railroad tracks and a parking lot separated the business district from a little park next to the river. "This is your 'great, good place,'" Burden continued, using a phrase from urban planning for a public place where people can gather and relax. "You would be honoring your great river if you moved the parking away from the shoreline and put it back in the street."

As he explained to his listeners, this morning's tour was the beginning of a process to rethink Muscatine's "built environment": the width of its streets, the length of its city blocks, whether there were trees downtown, how easily pedestrians could cross intersections. The goal was for participants to see their surroundings in a new way. Often, this was an eye-opening experience, even for longtime residents, Burden said. "People come up to me afterward and say, You know, I noticed things today that I've walked past a hundred times before. I don't think I'll ever walk by them again and not see them."

Just three months earlier, on January 30, 2013, we'd announced the selection of Muscatine as a new Blue Zones demonstration site—one of ten communities in Iowa with that designation. Over the next two years, our team of volunteers and staff would apply everything we'd learned in our Minnesota and California projects to launch a health revolution here in Muscatine and elsewhere in the state. Burden's walking workshop was an important part of that campaign, as were initiatives to transform smoking policies, strengthen social networks, and reshape the food environment.

One of the main reasons we'd picked Muscatine was the enthusiasm of its leadership. The individuals we'd met here had a clear sense of their town's identity and a determination to make it a better place to live. Under their stewardship, with partners in the business and philanthropic communities, the town had already increased its green space, expanded its bike trails, and created new routes for children to walk to school. But residents wanted more.

"Getting things like this done isn't easy," said Andrew Fangman, the city planner. "It takes commitment from public leaders and support from citizens. The Blue Zones program gives such efforts greater visibility. It moves things like walkability up in the community agenda."

We asked the team from the Gallup-Healthways Well-Being Index to do an initial assessment of where things stood in Muscatine. Based on their surveys, we discovered that the town's 23,000 or so residents weren't doing as well as the rest of Iowa when it came to life evaluation, emotional health, and physical health. When asked if they felt that their community "was getting better as a place to live," for example, residents responded with a score of 57.6 compared to Iowa's 60.8. When asked if they "ate healthy all day," they scored a 61.3 compared to Iowa's 65.8. Statistics for Muscatine County as a whole also raised a red flag, indicating that obesity, in both children and adults, was becoming a more serious problem.

PEARL OF THE MISSISSIPPI

That afternoon, at the town's History and Industry Center, Burden and I gave a short talk to introduce the Blue Zones Project to members of the public. All around us the small museum exhibits told the story of how Muscatine had earned the title "Pearl of the Mississippi." As it turns out, the name came from the button industry, which set up shop here in the 1880s. A German immigrant, J. F. Boepple, had founded the first company in town to make buttons from freshwater mussel shells taken from the Mississippi. Other companies followed. By 1915 Muscatine had won a reputation as the "pearl button capital of the world."

Today local businesses still upheld Muscatine's image as a mini-industrial center in the middle of farm country. Factories here made office furniture, herbicides, ketchup, animal feed, and lighting equipment for sports arenas, providing the community with a solid base of jobs and taxes. Yet Muscatine's leaders recognized that residents also wanted their community to become a healthier, more enjoyable place to live. And no one knew how to do that better than Burden.

"Every place I go to is different," he told the group at the museum. "But Iowa towns beautifully cluster into some commonalities. There's an agricultural base to many of the small communities. The streets of older ones are well connected, typically have good schools, active Main Streets—or at least you could tell that it was once active. Those foundations give us something to start with."

The problems in most towns began in the 1950s, he said, when Americans started building communities for cars instead of people. Streets got wider, speed limits got higher, and developers put in neighborhoods you had to drive to. "It was almost like somebody flipped a switch and we stopped building connected streets and started building disconnected ones like culs-de-sac—what I call 'dead worm' streets," Burden said. "I think we did that because of the economic engines at the time, which were busy building houses, filling those houses with appliances, building those roads, grabbing the cheap land, and getting more mortgages. But I believe that that era has drawn to a close. The big shift now is back to city centers to give people great places to live—and less time sitting in cars in frustration."

Research has shown that communities where it's easy to walk or ride a bike have lower rates of obesity, he said. Residents of such towns suffer less depression, have smaller carbon footprints, and enjoy higher property values. If traffic in your neighborhood is moving slowly, you tend to have up to three more friends on your block—and many more acquaintances—than people in neighborhoods with faster traffic. "If the speeds are low, you're out there walking, talking, meeting people," Burden said. "You might bump into somebody who tells you where to buy something. That person's not a friend, necessarily, just somebody you know because you had a conversation."

Making streets walkable is also good for business, Burden added. A few years ago, residents of a San Diego neighborhood asked him to help "calm down" the main thoroughfare in their business district. He suggested that they put the street on a "diet" by reducing the number of traffic lanes from five to two. That made room for curbside parking, bike lanes, a landscaped median, and safer pedestrian crossings. Foot traffic increased in the newly redesigned neighborhood, more businesses opened, and existing merchants reported a 30 percent boost in sales. Today that street, La Jolla Boulevard, is a model for urban planners.

"We can't afford to build places where people just park their bodies at night," Burden said. "We can't afford to spend a single transportation dollar that doesn't increase land value rather than decrease it." We should go back to building towns the way our great-grandparents did, he suggested. Most people today want to live in a community where they don't have to drive long distances. They want to live near enough to the stores and jobs so they can walk, take a bus, or ride a bike wherever they need to go.

If Muscatine wanted to stay competitive, retain existing businesses, attract new ones, and have money in the treasury for parks and other amenities, then the best thing residents could do would be to focus on making their town walkable and livable, Burden said. That meant adding sidewalks, improving crosswalks, replacing intersections with roundabouts in some places, and converting one-way streets to run in both directions.

"One-way streets help move people faster," Burden said. "But is that your goal? To empty out downtown?" You should be doing just the opposite, he argued. You want people to linger downtown and enjoy themselves. "Then, before you know it, your children won't be moving off to other cities. Everything they want will be right here in your own community."

As he always does, Burden got a rousing round of applause for his simple but powerful message. It was also a terrific pep talk for the people of Muscatine, as they prepared to launch their own Blue Zones revolution.

"Everything up to now has been practice," he told the group. "This is the one that matters."

LEARNING TO LISTEN

If you'd stopped by City Hall in Cedar Rapids on June 13, 2008, you'd have needed scuba gear to enter the conference room in the basement. The Cedar River, like many tributaries of the Mississippi that spring, had overflowed its banks, cresting at 19 feet above flood stage and submerging 10 square miles of the city. "It was a $6 billion disaster," said Mayor Ron Corbett, sitting in that same conference room today. "It was also a big emotional issue for our town. But like any town, people here wanted to come back. And they wanted to be better than they were before the disaster."

Since the floodwaters had receded, the city had invested more than $300 million in federal, state, and local funds to repair public facilities that had been damaged. Now 40 or so town leaders and city staff were gathered in the basement of City Hall to discuss a new phase of their town's development—participation in the Blue Zones demonstration project.

With a population of 128,000 or so, Cedar Rapids was by far the largest community we'd tackled so far. In practical terms, that meant we needed to account for a more diverse mix of stakeholders as we got the ball rolling here. For us, that translated into a lot of listening.

One way we did that was to hold charettes, or brainstorming sessions, to solicit ideas and opinions from residents. At one meeting, we helped a group put together a wish list of physical improvements, from new sidewalks and bike racks to a pedestrian bridge across the Cedar River. At another, we went over an extensive menu of policies related to food, such as creating a hub where small farmers could sell their produce to restaurants, schools, hospitals, institutions, and other food service establishments; or allowing vacant city-owned lots to be turned into community gardens; or loosening up regulations about chicken coops and beehives in city neighborhoods. After the group chose which policies would get the highest priority, our team helped them find sample policies, case studies, and other information about best practices.

The Soft Drinks Experiment

At first, the soft drink distributors didn't like the idea. As part of the Blue Zones Project in the town of Cedar Falls, the local Hy-Vee grocery store was considering an experiment to reduce sales of sugar-sweetened drinks and candy at its checkout counters, while boosting sales of healthier beverages and snacks. Was it possible to do this without making a dent in profits, the store managers wondered? The distributors figured they were all just going to lose business.

Eventually they agreed to work with the Hy-Vee staff to manage the test. The plan they decided on was to swap out two coolers that had been full of major-brand soda products. One got filled with Hy-Vee branded water and the other with national brands of bottled water, vitamin-enriched water, coconut water, and unsweetened tea. The store also replaced candy bars in checkout lanes with snack bars and baskets of fruit. Then they waited to see what would happen.

The results were impressive: After three months, the Cedar Falls Hy-Vee saw a 151 percent increase in healthy drink sales and a 99 percent increase in healthy snack bar sales. What nobody really expected, though, was an increase in *overall* sales of cold beverages. In fact, the Cedar Falls Hy-Vee was now outpacing all other midwestern locations in sales of water and noncarbonated beverages.

"This was one of our biggest successes," said Jeff Sesker, the Hy-Vee store director. He was proud of the leadership his store was taking on. "Sales of carbonated beverages have been declining nationally, but these figures indicate that Cedar Falls is ahead of the trend."

"Whatever we do, we need to let people have fun," Corbett said at one of these charettes. "People just need a little encouragement to participate in a healthy lifestyle." During the past year, he'd personally lost 25 pounds by exercising and eating better, he said. His cholesterol was also down. "I'm a big promoter of the Blue Zones," he added. "In a week and a half,

I'm going to run a half marathon, and I've been working hard for that. Two years ago I couldn't run a half mile."

But you don't have to run a half marathon to be a Blue Zones person, the mayor said. "Just take the first step," he suggested. "Take the first step and sign up for the pledge. Then take the next step."

GO RIDE A BIKE

There's nothing like a bike ride to clear your mind. At the end of our day in Cedar Rapids, I took a short drive into the Iowa countryside, unpacked a fold-up bicycle from my car and went out for a spin. The sun was just sinking behind the cornfields and the bovine bouquet wafting from nearby farms brought back fond memories of my Minnesota childhood.

Thinking back on the image of Knapp in the East Texas cotton fields, it occurred to me that there might be more similarities than I first realized between his campaign to modernize American farming and our own efforts here in Iowa to improve eating habits and encourage healthier lifestyles. At the time of his demonstration project in Terrell, the cost of food was a huge burden for American families, consuming 40 percent of their income, compared to less than 7 percent today. Farmers were stuck in the past, using outmoded techniques that produced low crop yields and exhausted the soil.

Today the deadweight around the necks of American families was the cost of health care. For every dollar we earn, we pay 18 cents in medical expenses, according to Atul Gawande, a Boston surgeon, who drew parallels between our health care and agricultural systems in a perceptive 2009 *New Yorker* article. As Gawande explained, part of our problem was that the current fee-for-service system offered all the wrong incentives. "It rewards doing more over doing right, it increases paperwork and the duplication of efforts, and it discourages clinicians from working together for the best possible results," he wrote. As a result, costs kept going up, but not the quality of medical care. "What have we gained by paying more than twice as much for medical care as we did a decade ago?" he asked.

I'd take this argument a step further and say that our whole approach to health today is backward. Instead of being designed around well-being, the economics are all lined up around sickness. Hospitals make money when you rent a bed and buy supplies. Doctors make money when you come in for a diagnosis and have tests. Pharmaceutical companies make money when you get sick and buy a prescription. But for the most part, nobody out there makes a profit by keeping you healthy.

That's what we were trying to change in Iowa—one demonstration town at a time. With the help of forward-thinking executives like John Forsyth at Wellmark Blue Cross and Blue Shield and Ben Leedle at Healthways, we were unleashing a swarm of Blue Zones ideas to give communities whatever they needed during the first three years of their effort to transform their environments for the long term and thrive. After all, nobody flipped a master switch to make farms more productive and food more affordable. It happened one farm at a time, with evidence-based advice from experts like Knapp. By 1930 the USDA had set up more than 750,000 demonstration farms across the nation.

Maybe we needed something like that to fix the health care system, Gawande suggested. The legislation behind Obamacare was packed full of Knapp-like pilot programs to reduce costs and improve results, including community wellness projects like our own. "Which of these programs will work?" he asked. "We can't know." It could take numerous different reforms and years of experimentation.

I'd suggest that it will take something else as well, something I'd underestimated at first in our community transformations. It was going to take a shift in local culture, a transformation of the way that people looked at their own communities. I'd seen it happen differently in each town. As residents embarked on Blue Zones initiatives—choosing healthier foods, adding trails and bike lanes, walking children to school, growing gardens, volunteering, discovering new purpose—they would stop at some point, look around, and say, Wow, we're becoming a healthy place.

That's how change was coming to Iowa. One town at a time. In the past, people might have said they were residents of the pork state. Now they said they were living in a Blue Zone.

MEASURES OF SUCCESS IN IOWA

Gallup's analysis found that Iowa Blue Zones Project communities showed statistically significant improvement between 2012 and 2013 in the following key areas of well-being:

- Nonsmoking improved by 8.8 percent
- Produce consumption improved by 10.5 percent
- Using strengths in workplace improved by 6.9 percent
- Enough money for food improved by 7.6 percent
- Health insurance improved by 6.0 percent
- Dentistry improved by 6.9 percent

During this time period Iowa communities that were not participating in the Blue Zones Project did not have statistically significant movement in these areas. At the same time, Iowa moved from #15 to #10 in Gallup's nationwide Well-Being rankings.

PART THREE

Building Your Own
Blue Zone

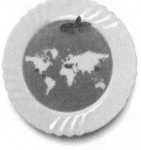

WHENEVER I SHARE WHAT WE'VE LEARNED in Blue Zones around the world—and how we're applying those same Blue Zones principles to transform communities in America—I see that look in people's eyes: They want to know how they can be part of it too. No one person can create a Blue Zone, of course, but one person—one family or one household—can take first steps in their own life by making small changes in what they eat and how they eat it. That's what this part of the book will share with you: lessons of Blue Zones eating that you can bring home.

CHAPTER TEN

❦

Food Rituals:
How to Eat to 100

A S WE'VE SEEN IN EVERY BLUE ZONE—both those around the world and those we're helping to shape here at home—food, diet, and eating habits are part of a much bigger picture. To understand our own habits, it first helps to step back and look at the wider cultural context that has shaped food choices and eating patterns here in the United States. First of all, you need to understand that if you're overweight, it's probably not your fault. We're hardwired by evolution to crave calories—delicious rich fat, glistening roasted meats, sweet foods, and carbs. For most of human history, those calories were extraordinarily hard to get. Our bodies hoarded calories to survive. When we indulge in high-fat, high-carb, high-salt foods, we're acting upon primeval organic impulses: to ingest as many calories as possible when they're available.

There was a time when this behavior promoted our species' survival, but things have changed dramatically in our food environment. Relatively recently in human history, refined starchy foods took the place of tubers and herbaceous plants in our diets. Sugar crept in. The quality and quantity of foods available changed drastically in the last few decades, with results at once triumphant and disastrous.

Some of the biggest changes came during the mid to late 20th century. Food science and government policy conspired to favor wheat, soybeans, sugar, and corn over other crops. Industrial agriculture increased productivity, even as small farms disappeared. Those few food crops predominated, and the food processing industry devised ways to use them to create cheaper food products that could be replicated in factories coast to coast and, ultimately, around the world. According to the USDA, from 1970 to 2000, the number of calories the average American consumed jumped by about 530 calories a day, a 24.5 percent increase. As food supply increased, food prices plummeted. At the beginning of the 20th century, we spent about 50 cents of every dollar earned on food; by the end of the century we were spending less than a dime of every dollar. Food companies, responding to demand, began engineering tastier processed foods, and they got very good at marketing them to us.

What makes it worse, at the same time that more food is so easily available, we've engineered physical activity out of our lives. There's a button to push for yard work, another for housework, and another to mix our food. An elevator takes us up three or four floors to the office. Our grandparents burned more than fives times as many calories in the regular daily activities of work and life, without resorting to "exercise." The number of miles the average American drives annually has nearly doubled, from 5,500 in 1970 to nearly 10,000 today.

If current trends continue, three-fourths of us will be overweight or obese and half of us will suffer from diabetes by 2030. The average American is already lugging 20 percent more weight than in 1970. Does that mean we're bad people? That we lack the discipline of our forefathers? Do we somehow care less about our health and our children's health than our grandparents did? No. Remember, we've gone from an environment of hardship and scarcity to one of abundance and ease. So if you're fat, it's probably not your fault. How do we overcome this?

The traditional answer has always had something to do with individual responsibility: Muster discipline and get on a diet and exercise program! The problem with that plan is that it requires long-term discipline and routine—both of which go against human nature. University of Minnesota professor Kathleen Vohs and her colleagues found that each morning we wake up with only a finite amount of discipline and once we deplete it, it's gone. We can use self-control for exercise, putting up with ornery kids, being nice to our spouse, trudging off to work, or avoiding those delicious calories. But at a certain point, the self-control bank account is empty. That's why we've designed the Blue Zones Solution to become a permanent part of your lifestyle.

MAKING FOOD AND DINING SACRED

Knowing which foods to eat—and in what quantities—is the first step toward eating to 100. But there's more that we can learn from people in the Blue Zones about the role of eating in the larger spheres of life. For them, growing, preparing, serving, and eating are all sacred practices with power to bring their families, their homes, their communities, their beliefs, and the natural world together in daily rhythms and harmonies. Centenarians in the Blue Zones follow daily rituals around food and meals. These rituals help them stay the course for the long run, and practicing them is certainly one of the keys to their longevity and sustained happiness with life.

After watching how Blue Zones principles can come to life in North American communities, I've settled in on six powerful food practices that create a virtuous circle between food, healthy social networks, moving naturally, strong spiritual life, and overall well-being. Here they are, along with a few thoughts on how to put them into practice in your own home.

Breakfast Like a King

There's an old saying: "Breakfast like a king; lunch like a prince; dinner like a pauper." In other words, make the first meal of your day the biggest, and eat only three meals per day. The routine is the same in almost all of the Blue Zones: People eat a huge breakfast before work, a medium-size late lunch, and a light, early dinner. They may occasionally grab a mid-morning piece of fruit or a mid-afternoon handful of nuts, but most don't make a habit of snacking. The average meal contains about 650 calories, so with just three meals a day, and a small snack, most people get all the calories a day they need. Adding a fourth meal, even a small one, can push your calorie consumption over the top for the day.

Most food is consumed before noon. Nicoyans often eat two breakfasts and a light dinner. Lunch tends to be the big meal for Ikarians and Sardinians. Okinawans like to skip dinner altogether. Many Adventists who follow the "breakfast-like-a-king" rule eat only two meals a day, one mid-morning and another around 4 p.m. There are a number of reasons this might help people live longer and lose weight.

Recent research supports front-loading calories early in the day. An Israeli study found that dieting women who ate half of their daily calories at breakfast, about a third at lunch, and a seventh at dinner lost an average of 19 pounds in 12 weeks. They also saw drops in triglycerides, glucose, insulin, and hormones that trigger hunger. Further, experiments with animals have confirmed that it's better not to skip breakfast: When lab rats were not fed before sleep and then starved for four hours after they awoke, they tended to overeat when finally given food. Other studies have shown that children who eat breakfast do better in school and are less likely to be overweight.

How you can do it:

- Make breakfast your biggest meal of the day. It should include protein, complex carbohydrates, and plant-based fats.
- Schedule breakfast early or as late as noon, depending on what works for your schedule.
- Expand your definition of breakfast beyond just cereal and eggs. In Nicoya, people add beans and corn tortillas; in Okinawa, it's miso soup; in Ikaria, it's bread and a bowl of savory beans.

Cook at Home

Cook your meals at home, and save eating out for celebrations. In most Blue Zones eating out is considered a celebratory field trip, a rare treat usually reserved for a wedding or other festive occasion. As globalization and the American food culture has encroached on the Blue Zones, restaurants too have been popping up in them (Ogimi, Okinawa, even boasts a longevity restaurant); but for the most part, people still eat at home and are likely the healthier for it.

When you cook at home, you can control the ingredients. You can choose the freshest, highest-quality ingredients and avoid consuming the cheap fillers and flavor enhancers that end up in much restaurant food. (Even high-end restaurants typically pile on the butter and salt.) Cooking also nudges you into action, requiring you to stand, stir, mix, knead, chop, and lift. All of this physical activity counts more than you know, especially when compared to sitting down at a restaurant.

Consider 80-year-old Eleni Kohilas of Raches Christos on Ikaria. I had the pleasure of watching her make bread one afternoon and realized at the time that I might have been witnessing the true explanation for why Ikarian sourdough bread contributes to longevity. The process started the night before baking day, when Kohilas walked to her neighbor's house to procure a marshmallow-size piece of sourdough. This exchange, of course, occasioned a half-hour conversation and a thorough download on the village gossip. After walking home, Kohilas mixed water, flour, and salt with the starter and kneaded the new dough for about a half hour—a full-body workout that engaged shoulder, arm, and core muscles. The following day Kohilas cut wood, stoked a fire in the outdoor oven, and tended the fire until it reached baking temperature. By lunchtime, she had six steaming loaves of healthy, delicious bread—and a two-hour workout under her belt. She'd burned enough calories making the bread to equal her first four pieces.

Now not everyone in North America is going to walk to a neighbor's house or build a fire to make a loaf of bread. But even making a simple meal in your kitchen could mean shaving 100 to 300 calories off your overall eating experience. Multiply those calories by 120—the number of times the average American eats out annually—and a new light shines on our obesity problem. One study followed the eating habits and caloric intake of 1,000 people for a week and discovered that, on average, people who ate out consumed about 275 more calories per day than people who ate at home. Why? Restaurants serve meals containing more calories. This may not sound like much, but by most estimates, just 200 extra calories per day could add up to as much as a 20-pound gain over the course of a year.

Finally, if you're cooking at home, you're likely to eat a narrower variety of foods in a single meal. The more items you are offered, the more food you tend to consume.

How you can do it:
- Always try to eat breakfast at home.
- Pack a lunch the night before.
- Prep ingredients for your dinner in the morning. Slow cooking is a great way to use your morning resolve to plan a Blue Zones dinner.
- Designate Sunday afternoon as your time to prepare meals for the week so that you can freeze food for later.

Hara Hachi Bu

In translation: Plan before you start eating to stop eating when you're 80 percent full. If you're ever lucky enough to share a meal with older Okinawans, as I have, you'll often see them murmuring these three words before they eat a meal. *Hara hachi bu* is a 2,500-year-old Confucian adage that reminds Okinawans to stop eating when their stomach is 80 percent full. Since it takes about 20 minutes for the feeling of fullness to travel from your stomach to your brain, this mnemonic device increases the likelihood that you will sense the growing fullness and stop eating before you are 100 percent full. Dietary expert Leslie Lytle has estimated that if the average American would follow the practice of hara hachi bu, he or she could lose 17 pounds in just the first year!

Perhaps even more important, rituals like hara hachi bu and other forms of saying grace also provides a pause in everyday living, forcing people to slow down and pay attention to their food. Ikarians, Sardinians, Costa Ricans, and Adventists all begin meals by saying a prayer. In many cases, these premeal rituals also remind people that food is special—it comes from an animal that give its life or is a gift of the land or a product of hard work. This sort of attention puts more value on food. Realizing that food is not just stuff to wolf down, but a blessing, something to be respected and praised, can change your relationship to food and the meals you share. Pausing before eating makes the meal a time to enjoy, relax, and release stress. As one Adventist preacher told me, "You're more likely to eat quality food if you express appreciation."

How you can do it:

- Try saying "hara hachi bu" as you begin meals or, if you are religiously inclined, say grace before meals. You can find your own way of doing this: Simply pausing for a moment of silence and saying or thinking what you feel is another way of recognizing the sacredness of your food.
- Wear a blue wristband. It may sound silly, but in doing so you will join with thousands of others in our Blue Zones cities across the continent. Throughout our projects we have distributed thousands of blue rubber bracelets to be used as a simple reminder to slow down at meals. Wear it—or your own version of it—for at least six weeks to enforce the habit. Research shows that if you can stick to a behavior for six weeks, you hit a tipping point that increases the chance it will become a permanent habit. Only things you do for a long time positively impact your life expectancy.
- Pre-plate food at the kitchen counter. People may eat up to 29 percent more when food is served family style. The trick is to serve food at the counter, put leftovers away *before* the meal, then serve plates on the table.

Fast Fasts

Learn the advantages of occasionally going without food. Fasting need not mean going for days without food and drink. As a matter of fact, you can experience the benefits of a small fast every 24 hours, by scheduling the time you eat during only 8 hours of the day. To do so, it's important to consume half of your day's calories at breakfast. It takes between 6 and 12 hours for our bodies to digest and absorb a meal. After this time, the body enters a fasting state, during which time it calls on reserves for energy—like stored fat—so establishing this schedule of eating 8 hours and fasting 16 can contribute to weight loss.

Other deliberate longer-term fasts are valuable as well. If you are religious, fasting may already be an important part of your practice. Greek Orthodox Ikarians fast up to half of the year, some days avoiding eggs and meat, other days avoiding food altogether. Devout Catholic Sardinians and Nicoyans fast during Lent, the 40 days before Easter, during which time they completely abstain from meat.

Recent scientific evidence shows that fasting, even for a day, can recalibrate insulin release, giving the pancreas a break. It can temporarily lower cholesterol and blood pressure. And fasting undeniably works as a short-term way to lose weight, break food addictions, and perhaps even cleanse the digestive tract. Most convincingly, moderate fasting for longer periods can create a form of caloric restriction and may slow aging.

Fasting puts the cells in our bodies into a survival mode, with at least two benefits. First, cells produce fewer free radicals, the oxidizing agents that "rust" our bodies from the inside out. Lower levels of free radicals strengthen arteries, brain cells, and even the skin. Second, occasional fasting seems to reduce levels of insulin-like growth factor 1 (IGF-1), a hormone important for cell growth in youth but potentially dangerous after about age 20, as high levels may promote prostate, breast, and other cancers.

Research also suggests that occasional fasting may stave off dementia. It keeps blood vessels healthy and may also spur brain cell growth, as shown in experiments with mice conducted by Mark P. Mattson, head of neuroscience at the National Institutes of Health.

How you can do it:
- If you belong to a faith, join other members of your faith during annual or weekly fasts. Religious fasts may be easier to adhere to than personal, solo fasts, since they are often reinforced by a social network and moral underpinnings.
- Find a "fast buddy." It's easier to fast with a friend.

- Limit food intake to 500 calories every other day to establish a regular fasting program and safely lose weight. With this and any other fasting program, drink six glasses of water daily.
- Try eating only two meals a day: a big late-morning brunch and a second meal at around 5 p.m.

IMPORTANT: Consult your doctor before fasting. Avoid starvation diets for more than a day at a time.

Eat With Friends and Family

Elevating the act of eating to a social event may help you enjoy and digest your food better by making your meals a time of sharing and being together with friends and family. I've eaten countless meals with people in the Blue Zones, and they were often three-hour affairs with a succession of many small plates punctuated by toasts, stories, jokes, and conversation. Mealtimes are celebrations, a time to give thanks, share stories, talk out problems, and bond as a family. Eating as a family forces you to slow down, making it less likely that you will overeat.

As a rule, people in the Blue Zones never eat alone, never eat standing up, and never eat with the other hand on the steering wheel. As my Ikarian guide Thea Parikos pointed out, when her family sits down to a meal, she leaves the stress hormones of the day elsewhere. Ikarians, she said, eat slowly while holding conversations with family, a ritual good for building not only stronger family ties but also healthier bodies.

How you eat can be as important as what you eat. If you eat on your feet and on the run, or driving in the car, stress hormones can interfere with your digestion and degrade food metabolism. Eating fast promotes overeating and, studies show, can double your risk of obesity. A 2011 study from the University of Illinois found that children and adolescents who share family meals three or more times per week are more likely to be in a normal weight range and have healthier dietary and eating patterns than those who share fewer family meals together. Other benefits include a reduction in likelihood of being overweight (12 percent), eating unhealthy foods (20 percent), and an increase in the likelihood of eating healthy foods (24 percent). Adolescents who eat dinner with their family are 15 percent less likely to become obese. Additionally, a report by the National Center on Addiction and Substance Abuse points out that teens who eat dinner with their family more than three times a week are less likely to do poorly in school. Make sure you have a comfortable kitchen table, ideally a round one, that is small enough to encourage family conversation.

How you can do it:
- Never eat standing up.
- Never eat while driving.
- When you eat alone, just eat. Avoid reading, watching TV, or perusing your phone or computer—all of which lead to faster, mindless eating.
- Establish a time and a family rule that everyone eats dinner together.

Celebrate and Enjoy Food

None of these rituals—nothing in the Blue Zones Solution—should feel like a restriction, a limitation, or deprivation. Don't deprive yourself. Go ahead and enjoy the good meals and the occasional indulgent celebration. We eat about 1,100 meals a year. If we celebrate a couple of times a week and enjoy what we love to eat, that still leaves almost 1,000 meals a year to eat the Blue Zones way.

"What dieters forget is that eating is one of the greatest pleasures of living," said Antonia Trichopoulou, arguably the greatest living expert on the Mediterranean diet. "Why would you want to miss any of this?" she asked, gesturing to the food on the table before us.

If they make you happy, you shouldn't give up that slice of pie at Thanksgiving, or that piece of birthday cake, or even that weekly steak. It may not be optimally healthy for you, but as residents of the Blue Zones have shown us, the body has some capacity to equalize after an occasional indulgence. The trick is painlessly finding that happy balance between savoring our lives and behaving in a way that saves them for the longest possible time. In our world, those two forces are at odds, but in the Blue Zones, those two forces harmonize.

How you can do it:
- Pick one day of the week and make it your celebratory day to splurge on a meal with your favorite foods. It could be Sunday after church or Saturday Sabbath, Monday to offset the beginning of the work-week, or Friday to celebrate another week well lived.
- Feel free to indulge at family celebrations and holidays. Find the individual balance that works for you.

Some of these Blue Zones food rituals will feel familiar to North Americans today. Eating one, two, and even three meals together as a family is part of our cultural tradition—but not necessarily part of our everyday lives anymore. On the other hand, some may seem new, even difficult. "Eighty percent full" in a culture of all-you-can-eat may mean a serious change in expectations. But after spending years watching these same food rituals mean so much to the centenarians I have met in every Blue Zone, I am sure they will benefit us too.

As will new lessons on just what to cook in the kitchen and serve at the table—which is what I'll be sharing in the rest of this chapter.

FOOD CHOICES FOR LONGEVITY

None of the Blue Zones centenarians I've ever met *tried* to live to 100. No one said at age 50, "You know what, I'm going to get on that longevity diet and live another 50 years!" They don't count calories, take vitamins, weigh protein grams, or even read labels. They don't restrict their food intake—in fact, they all celebrate with food. As we have applied the wisdom of the world's Blue Zones to transform cities in the United States, I've begun to believe that we can create the same sort of culture here.

It starts with food choices. Most of the Blue Zones residents I've come to know have easy access to locally sourced fruits and vegetables—largely pesticide free and organically raised. If not growing these food items in their own gardens, they have found places where they can purchase them, and more affordably than processed alternatives. They have incorporated certain nutritious foods into their daily or weekly meals—foods that often are not even found on the shelves of convenience stores or on the menus of fast-food restaurants across the country. They have inherited time-honored recipes or developed recipes on their own to make healthful foods taste good—a hugely important part of the picture, because if you don't like what you're eating, you're not going to eat it for very long.

The particular foods important to Blue Zones centenarians vary from one culture to the next. We have listed them at the end of each chapter in part I, and you will find them pulled together into one list on page 188. What may be just as important, though, are the

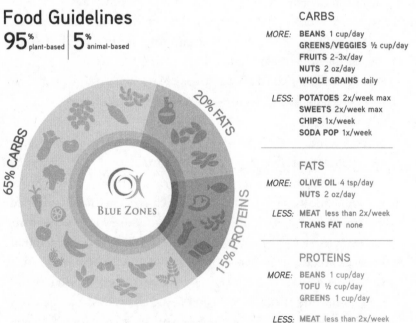

Food Guidelines
95%_{plant-based} | 5%_{animal-based}

CARBS

MORE: BEANS 1 cup/day
GREENS/VEGGIES ½ cup/day
FRUITS 2-3x/day
NUTS 2 oz/day
WHOLE GRAINS daily

LESS: POTATOES 2x/week max
SWEETS 2x/week max
CHIPS 1x/week
SODA POP 1x/week

FATS

MORE: OLIVE OIL 4 tsp/day
NUTS 2 oz/day

LESS: MEAT less than 2x/week
TRANS FAT none

PROTEINS

MORE: BEANS 1 cup/day
TOFU ½ cup/day
GREENS 1 cup/day

LESS: MEAT less than 2x/week
FISH 2x/week max
DAIRY

65% CARBS · 20% FATS · 15% PROTEINS

BLUE ZONES

guidelines for food selection that we have developed after visiting numerous Blue Zones and finding the best ways to translate those values for North Americans.

The findings here represent a long-term, statistical, and science-based study. We needed information that was not just anecdotal or based on interviews, visits in the kitchen, or shared meals with individual centenarians. We analyzed more than 150 dietary studies conducted in Blue Zones over the past century, and then we distilled those studies to arrive at a global average of what centenarians really ate. Here we provide some guidelines you can follow to eat like they do and live to 100.

BLUE ZONES FOOD GUIDELINES

Follow these guidelines and you'll crowd out refined starches and sugar, replace them with more wholesome, nutrient-dense, and fiber-rich foods—and do it all naturally.

1. PLANT SLANT See that 95 percent of your food comes from a plant or a plant product.

Limit animal protein in your diet to no more than one small serving per day. Favor beans, greens, yams and sweet potatoes, fruits, nuts, and seeds. Whole grains are okay too. While people in four of the five Blue Zones consume meat, they do so sparingly, using it as a celebratory food, a small side, or a way to flavor dishes. As our adviser Walter Willett of the Harvard School of Public Health puts it: "Meat is like radiation: We don't know the safe level." Indeed, research suggests that 30-year-old vegetarian Adventists will likely outlive their meat-eating counterparts by as many as eight years. At the same time, increasing the amount of plant-based foods in your meals has many salutary effects. In the Blue Zones people eat an impressive variety of garden vegetables when they are in season, and then they pickle or dry the surplus to enjoy during the off-season. The best of the best longevity foods are leafy greens such as spinach, kale, beet and turnip tops, chard, and collards. In Ikaria more than 75 varieties of edible greens grow like weeds; many contain ten times the polyphenols found in red wine. Studies have found that middle-aged people who consumed the equivalent of a cup of cooked greens daily *were half as likely to die* in the next four years as those who ate no greens.

Researchers have also found that people who consumed a quarter pound of fruit daily (about an apple) were 60 percent less likely to die during the next four years than those who didn't.

Many oils derive from plants, and they are all preferable to animal-based fats. We cannot say that olive oil is the only healthy plant-based oil, but it is the one most often used in the Blue Zones. Evidence shows that olive oil consumption increases good cholesterol and lowers bad cholesterol. In Ikaria we found that for middle-aged people about six tablespoons of olive oil daily seemed to cut the risk of dying in half. Combined with seasonal fruits and vegetables, whole grains and beans dominate Blue Zones meals all year long.

How you can do it:

- Keep your favorite fruits and vegetables on hand. Don't try to force yourself to eat ones you don't like. That may work for a while, but sooner or later it will fizzle. Try a variety of fruits and vegetables; know which ones you like, and keep your kitchen stocked with them. If you don't have access to fresh, affordable vegetables, frozen veggies are just fine. (In fact, they often have more nutrients in them since they're flash-frozen at the time of harvest rather than traveling for weeks to your local grocer's shelves.)
- Use olive oil like butter. Sauté vegetables over low heat in olive oil. You can also finish steamed or boiled vegetables by drizzling over them a little extra-virgin olive oil, which you should keep on your table.
- Stock up on whole grains. We found that oats, barley, brown rice, and ground corn figured into Blue Zones diets around the world. Wheat did not play as big a role in these cultures, and the grains they used contained less gluten than do the modern strains of today.

- Use whatever vegetables are going unused in your fridge to make vegetable soup by chopping them, browning them in olive oil and herbs, and adding boiling water to cover. Simmer until the vegetables are cooked and then season to taste. Freeze what you don't eat now in single or family-size containers, then serve later in the week or month when you don't have time to cook.

Notes on Protein

We've all been taught that our bodies need protein for strong bones and muscle development—but what's the right amount? The average American woman consumes 70 grams of protein daily, the average man more than 100 grams: Too much. The Centers for Disease Control and Prevention recommends 46 to 56 grams per day.

But quantity isn't all that matters. We also need the right *kind* of protein. Protein—also known as amino acids—comes in 21 varieties. Of those, the body can't make nine, which are called the nine "essential" amino acids because we need them and must get them from our diet. Meat and eggs will provide all nine amino acids while few plant food sources do. But meat and eggs also deliver fat and cholesterol, which tend to promote heart disease and cancer. So if you want to eat the Blue Zones way and emphasize plant-based foods, how do you do it? The trick is "pairing" certain foods together. By combining the right plant foods, you will get all the essential amino acids. You'll not only meet your protein needs but also keep your calorie intake in check.

2. RETREAT FROM MEAT Consume meat no more than twice a week.

Eat meat twice a week or even less in servings sized no more than two ounces cooked. Favor true free-range chicken and family-farmed pork or lamb instead of meats raised industrially. *Avoid* processed meats like hot dogs, luncheon meats, or sausages.

In most Blue Zones people ate small amounts of pork, chicken, or lamb. (Adventists, the one exception, ate no meat at all.) Families traditionally slaughtered their pig or goat for festival celebrations, ate heartily, and

PERFECT PROTEIN PAIRINGS

Peter J. Woolf, a chemical engineer and former assistant professor at the University of Michigan, worked with fellow researchers and analyzed more than 100 plant-based foods to identify the pairings and ratios that most efficiently meet our protein needs. Here are some of our favorite Blue Zones food pairings.

Quick and Easy Snacks

- 1½ cups cooked edamame sprinkled with soy sauce
- ¼ cup walnuts plus 1½ cups cooked edamame

Low-Calorie Combos

- 1⅓ cups chopped red peppers plus 3 cups cooked cauliflower
- 2 cups chopped carrots plus 1 cup cooked lentils
- 3 cups cooked mustard greens plus 1 cup cooked chickpeas
- 2 cups cooked carrots plus 1 cup lima beans
- 1 cup cooked black-eyed peas plus 1¼ cup cooked sweet yellow corn

Extra-Filling Dishes

- 1¼ cups cooked brown rice plus 1 cup cooked chickpeas
- 1½ cups cooked broccoli rabe plus 1⅓ cup cooked wild rice
- ⅔ cup extra firm tofu plus 1 cup cooked brown rice
- ½ cup firm tofu plus 1¼ cup cooked soba noodles

preserved the leftovers, which they would then use sparingly as fat for frying or as a condiment for flavor. Chickens roamed on the land, eating grubs and roosting freely. But chicken meat, likewise, was a rare treat savored over many meals.

Averaging out meat consumption over all Blue Zones, we found that people were eating small amounts of meat, about two ounces or less at a time, about *five times per month*. About once a month they splurged, usually on roasted pig or goat. Neither beef nor turkey figures significantly into the average Blue Zones diet.

Free-Range Meats

The meat people in the Blue Zones eat comes from free-roaming animals. These animals are not dosed with hormones, pesticides, or antibiotics and do not experience the misery of big feedlots. Goats graze continually on grasses, foliage, and herbs. Sardinian and Ikarian pigs eat kitchen scraps and forage for wild acorns and roots. These traditional husbandry practices likely produce meat with higher levels of healthy omega-3 fatty acids than the rich meat of grain-fed animals.

Moreover, we're not sure if people lived longer because they ate a little bit of meat or if they thrived *despite* it. There are so many healthy practices Blue Zones people engaged in, they may have been able to get away with a little meat now and then because its deleterious effect was counterbalanced by other food and lifestyle choices. As my friend Dean Ornish puts it, "The more healthier practices you undertake, the healthier you become."

How you can do it:

- Learn what two ounces of meat cooked looks like: **Chicken—** about half of a chicken breast fillet or the meat (not skin) of a chicken leg; **Pork or lamb—**a chop or slice the size of a deck of cards *before* cooking.
- Avoid bringing beef, hot dogs, luncheon meats, sausages, or other processed meats into your house.
- Find plant-based substitutes for the meat Americans are used to having at the center of a meal. Try lightly sautéed tofu, drizzled with olive oil; tempeh, another soy product; or black bean or chickpea cakes.
- Designate two days a week when you eat meat or other animal-derived food—and enjoy it only on those days.
- Since restaurant meat portions are almost always four ounces or more, split meat entrées with another person or ask ahead of time for a container to take half the meat portion home for later.

3. FISH IS FINE Eat up to three ounces of fish daily.
Think of three ounces as about the size of a deck of cards before it is cooked. Select fish that are common and abundant, not threatened by overfishing. The Adventist Health Study 2, which has been following 96,000 Americans since 2002, found that the people who lived the longest were not vegans or meat-eaters. They were "pesco-vegetarians," or pescatarians, people who ate a plant-based diet including a small portion of fish, up to once daily. In other Blue Zones, fish was a common part of everyday meals, eaten on average two to three times a week.

There are other ethical and health considerations involved in including fish in your diet. In the world's Blue Zones, in most cases, the fish being eaten are small, relatively inexpensive fish such as sardines, anchovies, and cod—middle-of-the-food-chain species that are not exposed to the high levels of mercury or other chemicals like PCBs that pollute our gourmet fish supply today. People in the Blue Zones don't overfish the waters as corporate fisheries do, threatening to deplete entire species. Blue Zones fishermen cannot afford to wreak havoc on the ecosystems they depend on. There is no Blue Zones evidence favoring any particular fish, though, including salmon.

How you can do it:
- Learn what three ounces looks like, whether it's three ounces of a larger fish such as snapper or trout or three ounces of smaller fish such as sardines or anchovies.
- Favor mid-chain fish like trout, snapper, grouper, sardines, and anchovies. Avoid predator fish like swordfish, shark, or tuna. Avoid overfished species like Chilean sea bass.
- Steer clear of "farmed" fish, as they are typically raised in over-crowded pens that make it necessary to use antibiotics, pesticides, and coloring.

4. DIMINISH DAIRY Minimize your consumption of cow's milk and dairy products such as cheese, cream, and butter.
Cow's milk does not figure significantly in any Blue Zones diet except that of the Adventists, some of whom eat eggs and dairy products. In

terms of the human diet, dairy is a relative newcomer, introduced about 8,000 to 10,000 years ago. Our digestive systems are not optimized for milk or milk products (other than human milk), and now we recognize that the number of people who (often unknowingly) have some difficulty digesting lactose may be as high as 60 percent.

Arguments against milk often focus on its high fat and sugar content. Neal Barnard, the founder and president of the Physicians Committee for Responsible Medicine, points out that 49 percent of the calories in whole milk and about 70 percent of the calories in cheese come from fat—and that much of this fat is saturated. All milk has lactose sugar as well. About 55 percent of the calories in skim milk come from lactose sugar, for example.

While Americans have relied on milk for calcium and protein for decades, people in the Blue Zones get these nutrients from plant-based sources. One cup of cooked kale or two-thirds of a cup of tofu, for instance, provides just as much bioavailable calcium as a cup of milk.

Small amounts of sheep's milk or goat's milk products—especially full-fat, naturally fermented yogurt with no added sugars—a few times weekly are okay. Goat's and sheep's milk products do figure prominently in the traditional menus of both the Ikarian and Sardinian Blue Zones. We don't know if it's the goat's milk or sheep's milk that makes people healthier or if it's the fact that people in the Blue Zones climb up and down the same hilly terrain as the goats. Interestingly, most goat's milk is consumed not as liquid but as fermented products such as yogurt, sour milk, or cheese. Although goat's milk contains lactose, it also contains lactase, an enzyme that helps the body digest lactose.

How you can do it:
- Try unsweetened soy, coconut, or almond milk as a dairy alternative. Most have as much protein as regular milk and often taste as good or better.
- Satisfy your occasional cheese cravings with cheese made from grass-fed goats or sheep. Try Sardinian pecorino Sardo or Greek feta. Both are rich, so you need only a small amount to flavor food.

5. OCCASIONAL EGG Eat no more than three eggs per week.

Eggs are consumed in all five Blue Zones, where people eat them an average of two to four times per week. As with meat protein, the egg is a side dish, eaten alongside a larger portion of a whole-grain or other plant-based feature. Nicoyans fry an egg to fold into a corn tortilla with a side of beans. Okinawans boil an egg in their soup. People in the Mediterranean Blue Zones fry an egg as a side dish with bread, almonds, and olives for breakfast.

Eggs in the Blue Zones come from chickens that range freely, eat a wide variety of natural foods, do not receive hormones or antibiotics, and produce slowly matured eggs that are naturally higher in omega-3 fatty acids. Factory-produced eggs come to maturity about twice as fast as eggs laid by breeds of chickens in the Blue Zones.

Eggs provide a complete protein that includes amino acids necessary for your body plus B vitamins, vitamins A, D, and E, and minerals such as selenium. Data from the Adventist Health Study 2 showed that egg-eating vegetarians lived slightly longer than vegans (though they tended to weigh more).

There are other health concerns that might influence your decision to eat eggs. Diabetics need to be cautious about consuming egg yolks, and egg consumption has been correlated to higher rates of prostate cancer for men and exacerbated kidney problems for women. Academics still argue about the effect of dietary cholesterol on arteries, but some people with heart or circulatory problems forgo them despite expert debate.

How you can do it:
- Buy only small eggs from cage-free, pastured chickens.
- Fill out a one-egg breakfast with fruit or other plant-based foods such as whole-grain porridge or bread.
- Try substituting scrambled tofu for eggs.
- In baking, use a quarter cup of applesauce, a quarter cup of mashed potatoes, or a small banana to substitute for one egg. There are also ways to use flax seeds or agar (extracted from algae) in recipes that call for eggs. Instructions for using these alternatives can be found online.

6. DAILY DOSE OF BEANS Eat at least a half cup of cooked beans daily.

Beans are the cornerstone of every Blue Zones diet in the world: black beans in Nicoya; lentils, garbanzo, and white beans in the Mediterranean; and soybeans in Okinawa. The long-lived populations in these Blue Zones eat at least four times as many beans as we do, on average. One five-country study, financed by the World Health Organization, found that eating 20 grams of beans daily reduced a person's risk of dying in any given year by about 8 percent.

The fact is, beans represent the consummate superfood. On average, they are made up of 21 percent protein, 77 percent complex carbohydrates (the kind that deliver a slow and steady energy, rather than the spike you get from refined carbohydrates like white flour), and only a few percent fat. They are also an excellent source of fiber. They're cheap and versatile, come in a variety of textures, and are packed with more nutrients per gram than any other food on Earth.

Humans have eaten beans for at least 8,000 years; they're part of our culinary DNA. Even the Bible's Book of Daniel (1:1-21) offers a two-week bean diet to make children healthier. The Blue Zones dietary average—at least a half cup per day—provides most of the vitamins and minerals you need. And because beans are so hearty and satisfying, they'll likely push less healthy foods out of your diet. Moreover, the high fiber content in beans helps healthy probiotics flourish in the gut.

How you can do it:

- Find ways to cook beans that taste good to you and your family. Centenarians in the Blue Zones know how to make beans taste good. If you don't have favorite recipes already, resolve to try three of the bean recipes in this book over the next month.
- Make sure your kitchen pantry has a variety of beans to prepare. Dry beans are cheapest, but canned beans are quicker. When buying canned beans, be sure to read the label: The only ingredients should be beans, water, spices, and perhaps a small amount of salt. Avoid the brands with added fat or sugar.

- Use pureed beans as a thickener to make soups creamy and protein-rich.
- Make salads heartier by sprinkling cooked beans onto them. Serve hummus or black bean cakes alongside salads for added texture and appeal.
- Keep your pantry stocked with condiments that dress up bean dishes and make them taste delicious. Mediterranean bean recipes, for example, usually include carrots, celery, and onion, seasoned with garlic, thyme, pepper, and bay leaves.
- When you go out to dinner, consider Mexican restaurants, which almost always serve pinto or black beans. Enhance the beans by adding rice, onions, peppers, guacamole, and hot sauce. Avoid white flour tortillas. Instead, opt for corn tortillas, with which beans are consumed in Costa Rica.

7. SLASH SUGAR Consume no more than seven added teaspoons a day.

Centenarians typically eat sweets only during celebrations. Their foods have no added sugar, and they typically sweeten their tea with honey. This adds up to about seven teaspoons of sugar a day. The lesson to us: Enjoy cookies, candy, and bakery items only a few times a week and ideally as part of a meal. Avoid foods with added sugar. Skip any product where sugar is among the first five ingredients listed. Limit sugar added to coffee, tea, or other foods to no more than four teaspoons per day. Break the habit of snacking on sugar-heavy sweets.

Let's face it: You can't avoid sugar. It occurs naturally in fruits, vegetables, and even milk. But that's not the problem. Between 1970 and 2000, the amount of added sugars in the food supply rose 25 percent. This adds up to about 22 teaspoons of added sugar that the average American consumes daily—insidious, hidden sugars mixed into sodas, yogurts, muffins, and sauces. Too much sugar in our diet has been shown to suppress the immune system, making it harder to fend off diseases. It also spikes insulin levels, which can lead to diabetes and lower fertility, make you fat, and even shorten your life. In the Blue

Zones, people consume about the same amount of naturally occurring sugars as North Americans do, but only about a fifth as much added sugar. The key: People in the Blue Zones consume sugar intentionally, not by habit or accident.

How you can do it:

- Make honey your go-to sweetener. Granted, honey spikes blood sugar levels just as sugar does, but it's harder to spoon in and doesn't dissolve as well in cold liquids. So, you tend to consume it more intentionally and consume less of it. Honey is a whole food product, and some honeys, like Ikarian heather honey, contain anti-inflammatory, anticancer, and antimicrobial properties.
- Avoid sugar-sweetened sodas, teas, and fruit drinks altogether. Sugar-sweetened soda is the single biggest source of added sugars in our diet—in fact, soft drink consumption may account for 50 percent of America's weight gain since 1970. One can of soda pop alone contains around ten teaspoons of sugar. If you must drink sodas, choose diet soda or, better yet, seltzer or sparkling water.
- Consume sweets as celebratory food. People in Blue Zones love sweets, but sweets (cookies, cakes, pies, desserts of many varieties) are almost always served as a celebratory food—after a Sunday meal, as part of a religious holiday, or during the village festivals. In fact, there are often special sweets for these special occasions. Limit desserts or treats to 100 calories. Eat just one serving a day or less.
- Consider fruit your sweet treat. Eat fresh fruit rather than dried fruit. Fresh fruit has more water and makes you feel fuller with fewer calories. In dried fruit, such as raisins and dates, the sugars are concentrated way beyond what you would get in a typical portion of the fruit when fresh.
- Watch out for processed foods with added sugar, particularly sauces, salad dressings, and ketchup. Many contain several teaspoons of added sugar.

- Watch for low-fat products, many of which are sugar-sweetened to make up for the lack of fat. Some low-fat yogurts, for instance, often contain more sugar—ounce for ounce—than soda pop.
- If your sweet tooth just won't quit, try stevia to sweeten your tea or coffee. It's not authentic Blue Zones, of course, but it's highly concentrated, so it's probably better than refined sugar.

8. SNACK ON NUTS Eat two handfuls of nuts per day.

A handful of nuts equals about two ounces, which appears to be the average amount that Blue Zones centenarians are eating. Almonds in Ikaria and Sardinia, pistachios in Nicoya, and all nuts with the Adventists—all nuts are good. Nut-eaters on average outlive non–nut-eaters by two to three years, according to the Adventist Health Study 2. Similarly, a recent Harvard study that followed 100,000 people for 30 years found that nut-eaters have a 20 percent lower mortality rate than non–nut-eaters. Other studies show that diets with nuts reduce "bad" LDL cholesterol by 9 percent to 20 percent, regardless of the amount of nuts consumed or the fat level in them. Other healthful ingredients in nuts include copper, fiber, folate, vitamin E, and arginine, an amino acid.

How you can do it:
- Keep nuts around your workplace for mid-morning or mid-afternoon snacks. Take small packages for travel and car trips.
- Try adding nuts or other seeds to salads and soups.
- Stock up on a variety of nuts. The optimal mix: almonds (high in vitamin E and magnesium), peanuts (high in protein and folate, a B vitamin), Brazil nuts (high in selenium, a mineral thought to possibly protect against prostate cancer), cashews (high in magnesium), and walnuts (high in alpha-linoleic acid, the only omega-3 fat found in a plant-based food). All of these nuts will help lower your cholesterol.
- Incorporate nuts into regular meals as a protein source.
- Eat some nuts before a meal to reduce the overall glycemic load.

9. SOUR ON BREAD Replace common bread with sourdough or 100 percent whole wheat bread.

Bread has been a staple in the human diet for at least 10,000 years. In three of the five Blue Zones, it is still a staple. While not typically used for sandwiches, it does make an appearance at most meals. But what people in Blue Zones are eating is a different food altogether from the bread that most North Americans buy. Most commercially available breads start with bleached white flour, which metabolizes quickly into sugar. White bread delivers relatively empty calories and spikes insulin levels. In fact, white bread (together with glucose) represents the standard glycemic index score of 100, against which all other foods are measured.

Refined flour is not the only problem inherent to our customary white or wheat breads. Gluten, a protein, gives bread its loft and texture, but it also creates digestive problems for some people. Bread in the Blue Zones is different: either whole grain or sourdough, each with its own healthful characteristics. Breads in Ikaria and Sardinia, for example, are made from a variety of 100 percent whole grains, including wheat, rye, and barley—each of which offer a wide spectrum of nutrients, such as tryptophan, an amino acid, and the minerals selenium and magnesium. Whole grains all have higher levels of fiber than most commonly used wheat flours. Interestingly, too, barley was the food most highly correlated with longevity in Sardinia.

Other traditional Blue Zones breads are made with naturally occurring bacteria called lactobacilli, which "digest" the starches and glutens while making the bread rise. The process also creates an acid—the "sour" in sourdough. The result is bread with less gluten than breads labeled "gluten-free" (and about one-thousandth the amount of gluten in normal breads), with a longer shelf life and a pleasantly sour taste that most people like. Most important, traditional sourdough breads actually *lower* the glycemic load of meals. That means they make your entire meal healthier, slower burning, easier on your pancreas, and more likely to make calories available as energy than stored as fat.

Be aware that commercial sourdough bread found in the grocery store can be very different from traditional, real sourdough, and thus may not have the same nutritional characteristics. If you want to buy true sourdough bread, shop from a reputable—probably local—bakery and ask them about their starter. A bakery that cannot answer that question is probably not making true sourdough bread.

How you can do it:

- If you're going to eat bread, be sure it's authentic sourdough bread like the ones they make in Ikaria. Sometimes called *pain au levain,* this slow-rising bread is made with lactobacteria as a rising agent, not commercial yeast.
- Try to make sourdough bread yourself, and make it from an authentic sourdough starter. Ed Wood, a fellow *National Geographic* writer, offers some of the best information on sourdough and starters at *sourdo.com.*
- Try a sprouted grain bread. When grains are sprouted, experts say, starches and proteins become easier to digest. Sprouted breads also offer more essential amino acids, minerals, and B vitamins than standard whole-grain varieties, and higher amounts of usable iron. Ounce for ounce, sprouts are thought to be among the most nutritious of foods.
- Choose whole-grain rye or pumpernickel bread over whole wheat: They have a lower glycemic index. But look at the label. Avoid rye breads that list wheat flour as their first ingredient and look for the bread that lists rye flour as the first ingredient. Most supermarket breads aren't true rye breads.
- Choose or make breads that incorporate seeds, nuts, dried fruits, and whole grains. A whole food (see the next Blue Zones food rule), like flaxseeds, adds flavor, complexity, texture, and nutritional value.
- Look for (or bake) coarse barley bread, with an average of 75 to 80 percent whole barley kernels.
- In general, if you can squeeze a slice of bread into a ball, it's the kind you should avoid. Look for heavy, dense, 100 percent whole-grain breads that are minimally processed.

10. GO WHOLLY WHOLE Eat foods that are recognizable for what they are.

Another definition of a "whole food" would be one that is made of a single ingredient, raw, cooked, ground, or fermented, and not highly processed. (Tofu is minimally processed, for example, while cheese doodles and frozen sausage dogs are highly processed.)

Throughout the world's Blue Zones, people traditionally eat the whole food. They don't throw the yolk away to make an egg-white omelet, or spin the fat out of their yogurt, or juice the fiber-rich pulp out of their fruits. They also don't enrich or add extra ingredients to change the nutritional profile of their foods. Instead of vitamins or other supplements, they get everything they need from nutrient-dense, fiber-rich whole foods. And when they prepare dishes, those dishes typically contain a half dozen or so ingredients, simply blended together.

Almost all of the food consumed by centenarians in the Blue Zones—up to 90 percent—also grows within a ten-mile radius of their home. Food preparation is simple. They eat raw fruits and vegetables; they grind whole grains themselves and then cook them slowly. They use fermentation—an ancient way to make nutrients bio-available—in the tofu, sourdough bread, wine, and pickled vegetables they eat.

Eating only whole foods, people living in the Blue Zones rarely ingest any artificial preservatives. The foods they eat, especially the grains, are digested slowly, so blood sugar doesn't spike. Nutritional scientists are only just beginning to understand how all the elements from the entire plant (rather than isolated nutrients) work together synergistically to bring forth ultimate health. There are likely many thousands of phytonutrients—naturally occurring nutritional components of plants—yet to be discovered.

How you can do it:

- Shop for foods at your local farmers markets or community-supported farms.
- Avoid factory-made foods.
- Avoid foods wrapped in plastic.

- Avoid food products made with more than five ingredients.
- Avoid premade or ready-to-eat meals.
- Try to eat at least three Super Blue Foods (see sidebar below) daily. You don't have to eat copious amounts of these foods. But you will likely discover that these foods go far to boost your energy and sense of vitality, so you'll be less likely to turn to the sugary, fatty, and processed stuff that gives you the immediate (and fast-fleeting) "fix."

A Blue Zones Beverage Rule

Drink coffee for breakfast, tea in the afternoon, wine at 5 p.m., and water all day. Never drink soda pop, including diet soda.

SUPER BLUE FOODS

Integrate at least three of these items into your daily diet to be sure you are eating plenty of whole food.

1. Beans—all kinds: black beans, pinto beans, garbanzo beans, black-eyed peas, lentils
2. Greens—spinach, kale, chards, beet tops, fennel tops
3. Sweet potatoes—don't confuse with yams.
4. Nuts—all kinds: almonds, peanuts, walnuts, sunflower seeds, Brazil nuts, cashews
5. Olive oil—green, extra-virgin is usually the best. Note that olive oil decomposes quickly, so buy no more than a month's supply at a time.
6. Oats—slow-cook or Irish steel-cut are best.
7. Barley—either in soups, as a hot cereal, or ground in bread
8. Fruits—all kinds
9. Green or herbal teas
10. Turmeric—as a spice or a tea

With very few exceptions, people in Blue Zones drank water, coffee, tea, and wine. Period. (Soda pop, which accounts for about half of America's sugar intake, was unknown to most Blue Zone centenarians.) There is a strong rationale for each.

WATER Adventists explicitly recommend seven glasses of water daily. They point to studies that show that being amply hydrated facilitates blood flow and lessens the chance of a blood clot. I feel that there is an added advantage: If people are drinking water, they're not drinking a sugar-laden beverage (soda, energy drinks, and fruit juices) or an artificially sweetened drink, many of which may be carcinogenic.

COFFEE Sardinians, Ikarians, and Nicoyans all drink copious amounts of coffee. Research findings associate coffee drinking with lower rates of dementia and Parkinson's disease. In addition, coffee tends to be shade-grown in the world's Blue Zones, a practice that benefits birds and the environment—another example of how Blue Zones eating practices reflect care for the bigger picture.

TEA People in all the Blue Zones drink tea. Okinawans nurse green tea all day long—and green tea has been shown to lower the risk of heart disease and several cancers. Ikarians drink brews of rosemary, wild sage, and dandelion—all herbs known to have anti-inflammatory properties.

RED WINE People who drink—in moderation—tend to outlive those who don't. (This doesn't mean you should start drinking if you don't drink now.) People in most Blue Zones drink one to three glasses of red wine per day, often with a meal and with friends. Wine has actually been found to help the system absorb plant-based antioxidants, so it especially complements a Blue Zones diet. These benefits may come from resveratrol, an antioxidant specific to red wine. But it may also be that a little alcohol at the end of the day reduces stress, which is good for overall health. In any case, more than two to three glasses a day for women and men, respectively, show adverse health effects. For women, there is also an increase in the risk of breast cancer with less than one drink per day.

How you can do it:

- Keep a full water bottle at your desk or place of work, and by your bed.
- Feel free to start the day with a cup of coffee. In the Blue Zones, coffee is lightly sweetened and drunk black without cream. Avoid coffee after mid-afternoon as caffeine can interfere with sleep (and, incidentally, centenarians sleep an average of eight hours nightly).
- Feel free to sip green tea all day; green tea usually contains about 25 percent as much caffeine as coffee and provides a steady stream of antioxidants.
- Try a variety of herbal teas, such as rosemary, oregano, or sage.
- Sweeten teas lightly with honey, and keep them in a pitcher in the fridge for easy access in hot weather.
- Never bring soda pop into your house.

DEVELOPING A TASTE FOR BLUE ZONES FOODS

If I've done my job so far, I've intrigued you with ideas on ways that you can nudge your own food choices toward those we found among people living in the Blue Zones. I've given you a list of foods that the world's longest-lived people eat, along with some guidelines on how to select, prepare, and eat them. Later in the book, I'll share recipes that go even further in helping you bring the foods from the Blue Zones into your kitchen and onto your table.

But what if you and your family don't like the foods on that list? I could tell you all day long that broccoli and beans are good for you. But if you hate broccoli and beans, you might eat them for a while, but you'll eventually tire of them and go back to eating what you're used to.

Almost everyone is born with a taste for sweetness and an aversion for bitterness. That's because, in general, sweetness means calories and bitterness sometimes signifies toxins. Early humans who gravitated toward the honey and berries were more likely to survive than those who nibbled bitter-tasting plants, even the greens that provided vitamins, minerals, and fiber. So we're naturally going to prefer candy bars over broccoli or brussels sprouts.

We're also born with our mother's tastes for certain foods. If our mothers ate salty foods high in saturated and trans-fats while they were pregnant with us, we're likely to be born with a taste for junk food. Conversely if a woman eats a lot of garlic prior to birth, the amniotic fluid will smell like garlic and the child will likely enjoy garlic. So, if your mom was not a healthy eater, as many mothers pregnant after 1950 weren't, you were probably born with a handicap.

Finally, most of our tastes are locked in at about age five. In fact, the sweet spot for acquiring new tastes is during the first year of life. Unfortunately most new mothers don't realize this, and they feed their kids porridge or sweetened baby food, which inclines the children's taste toward junk food for life. Or they give in to the convenience of buying their children salty, high-fat snacks. (French fries are the most commonly consumed vegetable for 15-month-olds in the United States.) In Blue Zones, mothers feed their babies many of the same whole foods they eat: rice, whole-grain porridge, and mashed-up fruits, for instance.

So what are the best ways to nudge yourself and your family toward the best choices, eating the Blue Zones way? To find out, I called Leann L. Birch of Penn State's Department of Nutritional Sciences and Marcia Pelchat of the Monell Chemical Senses Center in Philadelphia, who are both experts on acquiring tastes. I discovered that not only do we learn to like new foods throughout our lives, but there's actually a science-based strategy for learning to like the foods that are good for you. They gave me the basics for getting kids to like new, healthy foods such as vegetables. With small modification, these techniques will work for adults too.

How you can do it for kids:

- Kids are naturally wary of new foods, so prepare new vegetables with a texture familiar and appealing to your child. If he or she is used to pureed foods, start by offering new vegetables that are soft or can become soft when cooked. If your child likes crispy, crunchy food, then present new veggies raw.
- Introduce new foods when kids are hungry—before a meal or as a first course.
- Do not force foods on kids. You can turn them off for life.
- Introduce a variety of foods. Your kids may have a natural inclination toward peas and carrots but might hate broccoli and green beans. Serve small amounts of a half dozen vegetables at a time, a sort of Blue Zones succotash, and see which ones your kids like the best. Once you know that, you can try preparing those new favorites in different ways.

How you can do it for adults:

- Discover what you like. Take a cue from the notes above on how kids acquire tastes and try some new vegetables when you're hungry—as an appetizer before dinner, for example.
- Learn some new cooking skills. You're not going to eat vegetables unless you know how to prepare them in appealing ways. Recipes to start with—sure winners, as far as I am concerned—are Ikarian Stew (page 248), Sardinian minestrone from the Melis family (page 265), and Panchita's Gallo Pinto (page 291). We've taste tested these recipes as we have been doing Blue Zones community projects across the country, and we've found they appeal to thousands of Americans. The ingredients are cheap, the instructions are simple, and the results are delicious.
- Take a vegetarian cooking class.
- Host a Blue Zones potluck. Share the Blue Zones food rules and the list of ten Super Blue Foods (page 180) with a group of your friends. Ask everyone to bring a dish featuring one or some of those foods. You can all bring your culinary talents into play, trying new

plant-based foods, and also use them to strengthen your social network—a key goal of those who want to nudge their lives in the Blue Zones direction.

Four Always, Four to Avoid

It took a long time for my team to develop the ten Blue Zones food rules outlined above. And for some people, they may represent too drastic a change from the foods they have been eating all their lives. I understand—I was there too. When we first started working with the city of Albert Lea, I generally ate whatever was on hand. If my kitchen was stocked with ice cream and cookies, that was what I ate. I was a stalwart follower of the "See Food Diet": See food, eat it.

I knew we needed to start with some simple guidelines. I brought together some of the smartest people I could find, and we started by figuring out how to make kitchens healthier.

We reasoned that if we could identify the four best foods to always have on hand, and the four worst foods to never have on hand—and create a nudge—we might be able to get people to eat better. I included myself among the potential benefactors.

Cornell's Brian Wansink, the University of Minnesota's Leslie Lytle, and a few others got together to brainstorm the foods that were best and worst for us. We established a few criteria:

- The Always foods had to be readily available and affordable.
- The Always foods had to taste good and be versatile enough to include in most meals.
- The To Avoid foods had to be highly correlated with obesity, heart disease, or cancer as well as being a constant temptation in the average American diet.
- Strong evidence had to back up all food designations as Always and To Avoid.

Here's what we came up with and the thinking behind each decision.

Four Always

Remembering four food groups might be an easier starting point than remembering all the foods prepared in the Blue Zones. Here's our list.

100 PERCENT WHOLE WHEAT BREAD We figured it could be toasted in the morning and become part of a healthy sandwich at lunch. While not, perhaps, the perfect longevity food, it could help force white breads out of the diet and be an important step toward a healthier diet for most Americans.

NUTS We know that nut-eaters outlive those who don't eat nuts. Nuts come in a variety of flavors, and they're full of nutrients and healthy fat that satiate your appetite. The ideal snack is a two-ounce mix of nuts (about a handful). Ideally, you should keep small two-ounce packages on hand. Small quantities are best, since the oils in nuts degrade (oxidize). Larger quantities can be stored in the refrigerator or freezer for a couple of months.

BEANS I argue that beans of every type are the world's greatest longevity foods. They're cheap, versatile, and full of antioxidants, vitamins, and fiber, and they can be made to taste delicious. It's best to buy dry beans and it's easy to cook them, but low-sodium canned beans in non-BPA cans are okay too. Learn how to cook with beans and keep them on hand and you'll make a big leap toward living longer.

YOUR FAVORITE FRUIT Buy a beautiful fruit bowl, place it in the middle of your kitchen (either the counter, center island, or

FOUR ALWAYS	FOUR TO AVOID
100 percent whole wheat bread	Sugar-sweetened beverages
Nuts	Salty snacks
Beans	Processed meats
Fruits	Packaged sweets

table—wherever gets the most traffic), and place it under a light. Research shows that we really do eat what we see, so if chips are always in plain sight, that's what we'll eat. But if there is a fruit you like and keep in plain sight all the time, you'll eat more of it and be healthier for it. Don't bother buying a fruit you think you ought to eat but really don't like.

Four to Avoid

By the same token, remembering four rules that help you Blue Zone your refrigerator and kitchen cupboard might make the process easier. We're not saying that you can never treat yourself to these foods. In fact, if you love any of these foods and they make you happier, you should absolutely indulge occasionally. But save them for celebrations or, at the very least, make sure you have to go out to get them. Just don't bring them into your home, and you'll cut many of these toxic foods out of your diet without too much grief.

SUGAR-SWEETENED BEVERAGES Harvard's Willett has estimated that 50 percent of America's caloric gain is directly attributable to the empty calories and liquefied sugar that comes in sodas and boxed juices. Would you ever put ten teaspoons of sugar on your cereal? Probably not. But that's how much sugar you consume on average when you drink a 12-ounce can of soda pop.

SALTY SNACKS We spend about $6 billion a year on potato chips— the food (not coincidentally, perhaps) most highly correlated with obesity (though fried pork rinds are closing in fast). Almost all chips and crackers deliver high doses of salt, preservatives, and highly processed grains that quickly metabolize to sugar. They've also been carefully formulated to be optimally crunchy and tasty and to deliver a sultry mouth feel. In other words, they're engineered to be irresistible. So how do you resist them? Don't have them in your home!

PROCESSED MEATS A recent gold-standard epidemiology study followed more than half a million people for decades and found that those who consumed high amounts of sausages, salami, bacon, lunch meats, and other highly processed meats had the highest rates of cancers and heart disease. Again, the threat is twofold here. The nitrates and other preservatives used in these meat products are known carcinogens. They do the job, though, and preserve the products well, which means that processed meats are readily available on the shelf at home or in the store, right there for snacking or a quick meal.

PACKAGED SWEETS Like salty snacks, cookies, candy bars, muffins, granola bars, and even energy bars all deliver a punch of insulin-spiking sugars. We're all genetically hardwired to crave sweets, so we instinctively want to satiate a craving by ripping open a package of cookies and digging in. Lessons from the Blues Zones would tell us that if you want to bake some cookies or a cake and have it around, okay. If you want to enjoy the occasional baked treat at your corner bakery, fine. But don't stock your pantry with any wrapped sugary snacks.

For your convenience, I've brought together all the longevity foods into a single list, below. In the next part of the book, I'll share the best recipes I know that use these ingredients. Pick as many as you can, learn to prepare them, stick with them for the long run, and see how good they make you feel.

Longevity Superfoods From the World's Blue Zones

Vegetables

1. Fennel
2. Kombu (seaweed)
3. Wakame (seaweed)
4. Potatoes
5. Shiitake mushrooms
6. Squash

7. Sweet potatoes
8. Wild greens
9. Yams

Fruits

1. Avocados
2. Bananas
3. Bitter melons
4. Lemons
5. Papayas
6. *Pejivalles* (peach palms)
7. Plantains
8. Tomatoes

Beans (Legumes)

1. Black beans
2. Black-eyed peas
3. Chickpeas
4. Fava beans
5. Other cooked beans

Grains

1. Barley
2. Whole-grain bread
3. Brown rice
4. Maize *nixtamal*
5. Oatmeal

Nuts and Seeds

1. Almonds
2. Other nuts

Lean Protein

1. Salmon

2. Soy milk
3. Tofu

Dairy

1. Feta cheese
2. Pecorino cheese

Added Oils

1. Olive oil

Beverages

1. Coffee
2. Green tea
3. Red wine
4. Water

Sweeteners and Seasonings

1. Garlic
2. Honey
3. Mediterranean herbs
4. Milk thistle
5. Turmeric

But there is more to finding your own Blue Zones Solution than just picking and choosing from a list of foods. You need recipes, meal plans, and ideas on how to weave these foods into favorite recipes and prepare them so they taste like old familiars. That's what the rest of the book is meant to provide.

CHAPTER ELEVEN

✺

Blue Zones Menus: Meals and Snacks

P EOPLE IN THE BLUE ZONES DON'T JUST EAT TO LIVE, they also live to eat, and they eat for enjoyment as much as anyone else. As we look for ways to adapt their foods and customs to fit our own lifestyles, the idea isn't to kill the pleasures of eating but to crowd out the junk food from our daily routine with the foods the longest-lived people eat—and to enjoy doing it.

The inconvenient truth about longevity diets everywhere is that they contain fewer calories than we are used to eating. The average American woman consumes about 2,500 calories daily, the average American man about 3,200 calories. People in Blue Zones on average consume about 20 percent less: in other words, 2,000 calories for a woman and 2,560 calories for a man. So, you might ask, does eating fewer calories help explain longevity? Maybe. Apart from reducing the chances of being overweight or obese, eating less—caloric restriction, by its technical name—is the only proven way to slow aging in mammals.

Here's how it works: Inside our cells, as mitochondria convert food energy into the energy our bodies can use, free radicals exit the cells and circulate through the body, damaging arteries and organs including the brain, overstimulating the immune system, and causing inflammation, plaque buildup, and other problems. It's a process called oxidation, and it occurs inside the body much like rust deteriorates steel. When we mildly starve our cells of calories, though, the mitochondria kick into survival mode and throw off fewer free radicals, slowing the rust from within and reducing systemic inflammation. So as far as increased cellular damage causes aging, caloric restriction slows that process.

This is not a deprivation diet by any means, though. The goal is to feed your body the best way possible, and this meal plan will help you do it.

BLUE ZONES BREAKFAST

Plan your breakfast as the biggest meal of the day. Put together a hearty meal, using any of these four building blocks: (1) whole-grain cooked cereal, (2) Blue Zones smoothie, (3) beans, and (4) Blue Zones scramble.

Whole-Grain Cooked Cereal

I highly recommend a whole-grain cooked cereal as a foundation for your breakfast. I'm partial to whole-grain steel-cut oatmeal. (Not instant!) It's easy to mix and match ingredients to your taste and get all the carbohydrates, fats, and proteins in one bowl. Plus you can get oatmeal in most restaurants and hotels.

At home experiment with other whole-grain cooked cereals. Enjoy cooked brown rice exactly as you would a bowl of oatmeal, for instance. You can make a pot of brown rice at the beginning of the week and freeze it in portions to reheat with a little additional water or soy milk for breakfasts all week long.

Here is a list of additions:

- Chopped nuts of any kind. I recommend cooking them with the porridge rather than adding them at the end. Try macadamia nuts.
- Dried fruits—raisins or dates. All dried fruits are high in naturally occurring sugars. Cranberries, mangos, pineapples, and so on almost always have added sugars too.

- Peanut butter or other nut butters. Add one tablespoon.
- Ground flaxseed. Gives the oatmeal a nutty flavor and an omega-3 fatty-acid bump.
- Fresh fruit. Bananas, strawberries, and blueberries all work well.
- Coconut oil
- Cinnamon, pumpkin spice, or cardamom
- Plain soy, coconut, or almond milk. Use these instead of dairy milk, but read the label before you buy and avoid those that contain added sugars. I recommend you avoid dairy milk, cream, and butter.
- Sweeteners. Use a tablespoon or less of honey. Usually dried fruits, especially dates, will provide all the sweetening your cereal needs.

Blue Zones Smoothie

Use a blender or food processor to combine an assortment of nutritional and tasty ingredients for an easy breakfast meal in a glass. To get the carbs, proteins, and fats that make the most nutritional breakfast, smoothies should be made with a combination of fruits and vegetables, nuts or nut butter, and a liquid base. You can add certain ingredients to boost the fiber content, which makes the smoothie more filling. Don't use additional sweeteners. If you want your smoothies sweeter, add more banana to the recipe.

Experiment with fresh fruit and vegetable combinations to see what tastes best to you. Most fruit works, but I recommend either frozen fruit (easiest) or fresh fruit. Canned fruit often has added sugars. And while many have never considered vegetables a breakfast ingredient, adding greens to a smoothie is the best way to sneak them into your diet.

- Half a ripe banana
- Blueberries
- Strawberries
- Mango (Frozen are good and cheap.)
- Kale (fresh, cooked, or frozen)

- Spinach (fresh, cooked, or frozen)
- Broccoli (cooked or frozen)

A tablespoon of peanut butter, almond butter, or any other nut butter gives the smoothie protein and fat—hence the lasting power to fuel you through the morning.

Certain ingredients increase the fiber content and make you feel fuller. Add any one of the following:

- Raspberries or blackberries. One cup has eight grams of fiber.
- Ground flaxseed. Two tablespoons have four grams of fiber.
- Chia seeds. Half a tablespoon has about 5.5 grams of fiber. (But drink quickly! Chia seeds thicken your smoothie fast.)

Often the ingredients you put into a smoothie are thick, needing a liquid to lighten the drink. Consider using:

- Plain soy milk
- Almond milk
- Coconut milk
- Coconut water

Beans for Breakfast

While most of us aren't used to starting our day with beans, they are commonly found on the breakfast table in the Blue Zones. A cup of beans a day is the best longevity supplement available, so breakfast is your chance to get a head start on the daily quota.

Start with a serving of black or pinto beans, either homemade or from a can. (Read the label on canned beans to be sure you have chosen a brand without added sugar or fat.) Better yet, serve leftovers from a bean dish you cooked the day before.

Serve corn tortillas with simple cooked beans. Again, read the label: Look for whole-grain corn with no added ingredients except salt and water. Or serve rice with cooked beans for breakfast. Brown rice is best, but white rice is okay too, since the glycemic load of white rice drops into the safety zone when you eat it together with beans.

Blue Zones Scramble

Eggs are the centerpiece of many American breakfasts. But to follow a Blue Zones food plan, it's best to keep them at a minimum—no more than three per week. You can still cook protein-rich scrambled breakfast dishes, though, with other ingredients closer to what people eat for breakfast in the Blue Zones. Mince firm tofu and salmon, canned or fresh wild-caught, for an egg substitute or to extend one egg into more servings. Cook with olive or canola oil rather than butter. Stir in the vegetables—peppers, onions, spinach, broccoli, tomatoes, onions, spinach—season with plenty of spices, or fresh green herbs such as oregano, thyme, sage, and dill. Add a dash of Tabasco or other hot sauce, and you have a delicious, nutritious Blue Zones scramble.

A side serving of any sort of fresh fruit, including a fruit salad (hold the sugar) will go nicely with your scramble. We've been conditioned in America to drink fruit juice, but it doesn't figure prominently in a Blue Zones food plan. The fact is, fruit juices, even those without added sugar, have almost the same effect on your blood sugar as soda pop. So skip the fruit juice altogether and opt for the whole fruit instead. While whole fruit does contain sugar, its fiber offsets the sugar.

Toast, the perennial breakfast item, does not find its way into many Blue Zones breakfasts. Most breads available in the United States deliver too many simple carbs. But one toasted slice of true sourdough bread or true whole-grain bread, topped with nut butter or smashed avocado, would be fine.

Recipes for a Blue Zones Breakfast

Slow-Cooker Oatmeal *(Adventist)*, page 279
Homemade Granola *(Adventist)*, page 280
Ikarian Teas *(Ikaria)*, page 244

BLUE ZONES LUNCH

In the Blue Zones, the midday meal is typically consumed between noon and mid-afternoon, and it is usually the second largest meal of the day. It is often the meal that brings the family together. In America the lunch traditions are so different. Lunches are often eaten at school or at work from a Tupperware container, or they are eaten on the go. Few Americans will be able to adapt to a family meal in the middle of the day, so the lunch basics offered in this book translate Blue Zones eating practice into the American on-the-go lifestyle. And you don't have to cook something for a midday meal: The best lunches are often yesterday's dinner. Almost all Blue Zones dinner entrées can be prepared in advance or in extra portions and eaten, hot or cold, as lunches all week long. Many soups take time to prepare, but they can also be made ahead and frozen in single servings for a week of lunches.

The Sandwich

Millions of American think that lunch has to be a sandwich, but consider an open-face sandwich or an extra thick half sandwich, and choose your sandwich makings carefully.

Breads and Wraps
- Pumpernickel
- Real sourdough bread
- Sprouted grain bread
- Sprouted grain tortilla
- Whole-grain corn tortilla

Hearty Sandwich Center
- Hummus
- Salmon, smoked or canned
- Marinated tofu
- Tempeh

- Avocado
- Nut butters

Healthy Additions

- Sliced or grilled onion
- Sliced tomato
- Shredded lettuce or other fresh greens
- Sliced and pitted avocado
- Sun-dried tomatoes
- Sliced mushrooms
- Roasted red peppers
- Seasoned and sliced fresh or pickled jalapeño peppers
- Pickles
- Sliced, pitted olives
- Sliced cucumbers

Spreads

- Smashed avocado
- Mustard (Read the label when purchasing to avoid added sugar.)
- Regular or vegan mayonnaise
- Oil and vinegar salad dressing

Recipes for a Blue Zones Lunch

TLT on Toast *(Adventist)*, page 281

Melis Family Minestrone *(Sardinia)*, page 265

Minestra di Fagioli *(Sardinia)*, page 267

Lentil Soup, page 231

Miso Soup With Vegetables *(Okinawa)*, page 255

Creamy Squash and Bean Soup *(Nicoya)*, page 287

Easy Tomato Salsa *(Adventist)*, page 284

Tropical Cabbage Salad *(Nicoya)*, page 288

Gazpacho *(Nicoya)*, page 288

Avocado Salsa *(Adventist)*, page 284

White Bean Smash *(Sardinia),* page 270
Chickpea Hummus *(Sardinia),* page 271

BLUE ZONES DINNER

In the Blue Zones, the midday meal is the main meal of the day, while the evening meal is the smallest. The most complete Blue Zones food makeover would involve making this shift in the balance of meals, but our American culture puts a lot of emphasis on dinner as the largest, and often the most social, meal of the day. Instead of meat and potatoes, though, think beans and vegetables. There are plenty of meatless entrées that are tasty, filling, and nutritious, especially if you pay attention to protein pairings—food combinations that provide all the necessary amino acids (and plenty of fiber and nutrients) to round out your eating day.

Here are a few of the many combinations that represent complete protein pairings:

- 1⅓ cups chopped red peppers plus 3 cups cooked cauliflower
- 2 cups chopped carrots plus 1 cup cooked lentils
- 3 cups cooked mustard greens plus 1 cup cooked chickpeas
- 2 cups cooked carrots plus 1 cup cooked lima beans
- 1 cup cooked black-eyed peas plus 1¼ cup cooked sweet yellow corn
- 2 tablespoons "natural" peanut butter (made with just peanuts; no sugars or additives) plus 1 slice 100 percent whole wheat bread (stone-ground preferable)

And here are some protein pairings that include more carbohydrates, which makes them extra-filling:

- 1¼ cups cooked brown rice plus 1 cup cooked chickpeas
- 1½ cups cooked broccoli rabe plus 1⅓ cups cooked wild rice
- ⅔ cup extra firm tofu plus 1 cup cooked brown rice
- ½ cup firm tofu plus 1¼ cups cooked soba noodles

Making Vegetables Delicious

Next to beans, vegetables are the most important item to be added to the American diet in order to bring it more in line with the food traditions of centenarians in the Blue Zones. Unfortunately, many children and a lot of adults have developed an antipathy toward vegetables, so part of turning your home into a Blue Zone will be discovering ways to cook vegetables that make them irresistibly delicious.

One secret to making steamed or boiled vegetables taste delicious is to finish them with a drizzle of oil, salt, and the herb or spice of your choice, including black pepper, red pepper flakes, cumin, oregano, turmeric, thyme, or sage.

There are a number of other ways to combine, enhance, and prepare vegetables. Explore the possibilities to find out which works best for you and your family. Many Blue Zones vegetable recipes call for slow cooking over low heat for several hours—perfect for slow cookers. Slow cooking not only helps prevent nutrient breakdown but also blends and intensifies flavors. Frying foods at high temperatures breaks down oils and, in some cases, creates toxins. As a rule, you don't want oil to get so hot it smokes. (Olive oil smokes at 325 to 375 degrees; canola oil at 425 to 475 degrees.) If you want to quick-cook vegetables by frying, it's better to stir-fry or sauté foods at medium heat. It takes slightly longer, but the result is much healthier and often tastier.

Recipes for Blue Zones Vegetable Dishes

Thea's Greek Salad *(Ikaria)*, page 245
Horta – Longevity Greens *(Ikaria)*, page 246
Horta With a Fried Egg *(Ikaria)*, page 247
Greek Potato Salad *(Ikaria)*, page 247
Fava Bean and Mint Salad *(Sardinia)*, page 268
Tomato, Artichoke, and Fennel Salad *(Sardinia)*, page 269
Marinated Antipasto *(Adventist)*, page 282
Quinoa Salad With Sweet Potatoes and Pears *(Adventist)*, page 283
Sardinian Tomato Sauce *(Sardinia)*, page 270

Easy Tomato Salsa *(Adventist)*, page 284
Tropical Cabbage Salad *(Nicoya)*, page 288
Gazpacho *(Nicoya)*, page 288
Avocado Salsa *(Adventist)*, page 284
White Bean Smash *(Sardinia)*, page 270
Chickpea Hummus *(Sardinia)*, page 271
Stuffed Acorn Squash *(Adventist)*, page 285
Vegetarian Stuffed Bells *(Adventist)*, page 286
Coconut-Mashed Sweet Potatoes *(Okinawa)*, page 256
"Stone"-Baked Sweet Potatoes *(Okinawa)*, page 257
Somen Noodles With Steamed Vegetables *(Okinawa)*, page 257
Plantains Two Ways *(Nicoya)*, page 289
Toasted Spiced Chickpeas *(Sardinia)*, page 271

MAKING THE BEST OF BEANS

I argue that the world's best longevity supplement is a cup of beans per day. We don't know exactly why people in Blue Zones live such a long time, but it may be because they eat beans daily instead of meat—and the people I have met in the Blue Zones certainly know how to make beans taste good.

Unfortunately, beans come with a bad reputation. They're rich in oligosaccharides, very complex carbohydrates that cannot be digested by enzymes found in the gut alone, so they continue to be broken down in the intestines by a process called bacterial fermentation. In other words, the gas that comes as a result of eating cooked beans is the product of millions of tiny bacterial farts. The more you eat beans, the better your gut is in digesting them, but here are some tips on preparing beans to reduce bacterial formation:

- Favor pinto beans, black beans, black-eyed peas, mung beans, adzuki beans, and lentils, as they are easier to digest. Kidney beans, fava beans, and navy beans are harder to digest and thus likely to give rise to more gas.

- Add a teaspoon of baking soda to the water while soaking beans before cooking them.
- Add turmeric, ginger, or fennel: All seem to help process the complex carbohydrates. Other herbs and spices help too.
- Eat sliced oranges as a side to your beans. Many people find this helpful.
- Eat more beans. Most experts agree gas problems diminish or disappear with regular bean consumption.

But if you don't like beans, you won't eat them. The best way to get to know them is to cook them using recipes from those who know them well.

Recipes for Beans From the Blue Zones

Lentil Soup, page 231
Creamy Squash and Bean Soup *(Nicoya)*, page 287
Fava Bean and Mint Salad *(Sardinia)*, page 268
White Bean Smash *(Sardinia)*, page 270
Chickpea Hummus *(Sardinia)*, page 271
Panchita's Gallo Pinto *(Nicoya)*, page 291
Gallo Pinto With Salsa Lizano *(Nicoya)*, page 291
Bean and Squash Tortillas With Papaya Salsa *(Nicoya)*, page 293
Tropical Lentil Stew *(Nicoya)*, page 294
Basic Cooked Beans, page 233
Lia's Black Beans, page 241
Black Bean Soup, page 234
Mark Bittman's Chili Non Carne, page 243
Brenda's Maple-Ginger Red Beans, page 240
Spicy Bean Burgers, page 235
Slow-Cooked Vegetarian Black Bean and Potato Stew, page 236
Michele Scicolone's Giant Beans in Tomato Sauce, page 241
White Bean and Root Vegetable Casserole, page 237
Spiced Lentils, page 232

QUICK AND EASY SNACKS THE BLUE ZONES WAY

I have found that centenarians in the Blue Zones generally do not eat snacks. They are satisfied with the meals they prepare and move on to other activities between meals. Americans love their snack foods, though, and snacks are likely the place where we tend to give in to the urge to eat highly sweetened or salty processed foods, generally high in calories but low in nutritional value. Take some ideas from the list of Blue Zones foods and change your family's snacking habits, offering, for instance, nuts, fruit (except grapes, which are high in sugar), or cooked edamame (green soybeans) sprinkled with soy sauce.

Recipes for Blue Zones Snacks

Easy Tomato Salsa *(Adventist)*, page 284
Avocado Salsa *(Adventist)*, page 284
White Bean Smash *(Sardinia)*, page 270
Chickpea Hummus *(Sardinia)*, page 271
Plantains Patacones Style *(Nicoya)*, page 290
Sweet Plantains *(Nicoya)*, page 290
Toasted Spiced Chickpeas *(Sardinia)*, page 271

CELEBRATORY FOOD

Blue Zones centenarians tend to eat dishes with meat—usually pork or chicken—only once a week or even less. To them, a meat-enhanced entrée is a special treat, and meat-based foods that we might consider dinner entrées in the United States would be considered special celebratory foods. As you transition your meals and menu toward the Blue Zones food plan, you will find yourself eating meat less often, saving it for special occasions, and using a smaller amount as flavoring rather than considering it a dish in itself.

Recipes for Blue Zones Celebratory Meals

Goya Champuru—Bitter Melon Stir Fry *(Okinawa),* page 261

Shoyu Pork *(Okinawa),* page 263

Yakisoba *(Okinawa),* page 264

Blue Zones Pork and Beans, page 238

Rotelle With Chopped Pork and Tomato *(Sardinia),* page 278

Favata *(Sardinia),* page 275

Picadillo With Mango and Pork *(Nicoya),* page 295

Pane Frattau *(Sardinia),* page 276

Roasted Sardines *(Sardinia),* page 277

Pollo Guisado *(Nicoya),* page 296

Mark Bittman's Stewed Chickpeas With Chicken, page 242

These new foods and food rules may seem like a lot of changes to navigate. The important thing is to take it slowly, step-by-step, and nudge yourself and your family into new eating practices. It's just as important to be aware of how your eating and lifestyle habits are shaped by your home and community. To change health behaviors for the long run, you have to know the right things to do, have practical advice on how do them, and set up your environment so they are easy to do. The next chapter will show you how to set up you surroundings so you are doing what you can to make your home a Blue Zone.

CHAPTER TWELVE

꩜

Blue Zones Living: A Design for Easy Health

NOW YOU KNOW WHAT PEOPLE who live to 100 eat and the daily rituals that link their food to a virtuous web of healthy living. This chapter is about setting up your own surroundings so that healthy Blue Zones choices are always the easiest ones. If you're an American, you live within a mile of an average of seven fast-food restaurants, and you're barraged with offers of cheap, empty calories all day long. How do you beat back this temptation? Our society has engineered much of daily movement out of our lives. TVs, computers, and handheld devices isolate us from face-to-face human contact. How can you curate your surroundings to build your personal Blue Zone?

Remember, the longevity all-stars from the Blue Zones don't rely on day-to-day behavioral change. Longevity happens to them. As we've seen, they live in places where the healthiest foods are the most accessible. But they also move all day long. In America we don't. The average American sits 9.6 hours a day. For every hour we sit, we lose about 22 minutes of life expectancy. After just the first seated hour, fat-burning hormones in our blood significantly decrease.

Taking a closer look at the lives and environment of Blue Zones residents can give us a good idea of how to set up our own homes. I estimate that in Blue Zones, people are nudged into some form of physical activity—gardening, food preparation, cleaning, walking, or just getting up off the floor—every 10 to 15 minutes. They maintain a high metabolism all day long, every day. In Nicoya women still grind corn and pat tortillas by hand. In Ikaria they knead bread. In Okinawa houses are almost devoid of furniture, so Okinawans get up and down from the floor dozens of times every day—even into their 90s and 100s.

This physical activity counts! And it arguably counts more than going to the gym for an hour at day's end. Why? Because after about 90 minutes of sitting, your body drops into sort of a hibernation state. In this state, calories you consumed during your last meal are more likely to end up as stored fat around your waist than as fuel to boost your energy level. But if you live in a home that is full of nudges that keep you moving, you're not only burning more calories with physical activity, you're also keeping your metabolism working at a higher rate. This natural movement creates a heart-healthy, fat-burning blood chemistry that keeps you sharper and feeling more energetic.

On average, centenarians report sleeping about eight hours per day. Research has shown that when people get less than seven hours of sleep per night, their chance of catching a cold triples, they report as much as 30 percent lower rates of well-being, their risk of obesity soars, and they have less control over their hunger urges. So setting up the proper sleep environment sets up the rest of the day.

People in Blue Zones suffer from the same stresses that we do. They worry about their kids, their money, and their health. What they have that many Americans don't are sacred daily rituals that help them downshift—and reverse the stress of daily living. This is important because stress triggers inflammation, and chronic inflammation is at the root of every age-related disease, including heart disease, some cancers, and even Alzheimer's disease. You can't escape stress altogether, but you can set up your surroundings so you have less of it.

There is a burgeoning body of research showing that we can make long-term changes to our personal environment that nudge us into moving more, socializing more, eating less, and eating better. In other words, you can make a number of decisions right now that will lead you to a healthier, happier future. When it comes to living longer, there's no short-term fix. Ubiquitous, long-lasting tweaks to your environment will add up to big changes in the rest of your life.

From the kitchen to your bedroom, into the yard and out into your community, here are some changes you can make right now to create your own Blue Zone.

BLUE ZONE YOUR KITCHEN

There are four simple things you can do to create your own Blue Zones kitchen. First, keep the healthiest ingredients on hand and in plain sight. Second, equip your kitchen with cookware and utensils that enable you to make delicious Blue Zones foods quickly. Third, keep safety your top priority. And fourth, develop the habit of using nonmechanized appliances to keep you moving naturally while you cook.

Blue Zones kitchens around the world are stocked with hand-operated equipment that makes preparing and cooking food a more physical and meditative process. Many aspects of your kitchen, large and small, can be set up to encourage you to prepare and serve great food. You don't need expensive new equipment or state-of-the-art appliances to cook the Blue Zones way. (Remember the dented pans in Athina Mazari's Ikarian kitchen?)

Here are the most important considerations:

LAYOUT The most efficient kitchens are set up as a triangle, with the stove, sink, and refrigerator each a point of the triangle. Ideally, the sink sits next to the stove on one side and the refrigerator on the other. This layout optimizes efficiency and will help make cooking more enjoyable. Some kitchens, such as an apartment galley kitchen, might not have the depth for a true triangle. In that case, the stove, sink, and fridge should line up, in that order. The garbage can should also be within easy reach. Even if your kitchen is not designed in this triangle of efficiency, think about your workflow and access patterns, positioning movable things such as cutting boards, hanging equipment, and flatware where most convenient.

THE RIGHT REFRIGERATOR A newer, smaller refrigerator may be a good health investment. Why newer? Because the latest models keep fruit, vegetables, and other food fresh longer by eliminating bacteria and gases more efficiently, thus hindering spoilage. Unfortunately, the nutrient quality of fruits and vegetables begins to degrade as soon as they are picked. And why smaller? Recent studies have shown that the more food in your refrigerator, the more you're likely to eat. So a small refrigerator can serve as a nudge to eat less. A smaller refrigerator will also get you out of the house more often—perhaps even daily, as we see in Blue Zones—to go shopping for fresh foods.

PLENTY OF CLEARED COUNTER SPACE You will feel best about cooking if you have a large, inviting space on which to chop and prepare your food. (Put your TV and mail elsewhere.)

GOOD LIGHTING To enjoy preparing food, make sure your prep space has plenty of light. Most people find warm, incandescent bulbs more pleasant than fluorescent lights. Eyestrain can be a negative nudge, subconsciously driving you away from cooking.

SMALL PANTRY Our grandparents used pantries to store homemade conserves, pickled vegetables, and fruit jams; today's pantries are more likely to carry gigantic bags of chips and pretzels, cases of granola bars, and boxes of cereal—large quantities of packaged food, bought because the price was so low. But one study found that people prepared 23 percent more food when cooking from large containers—a good reason to leave the 25-pound bag of rice at the supermarket.

THE RIGHT EQUIPMENT Certain implements become essential as you make the transition from electric appliances.

- *Solid cutting board.* You want one that won't crack or warp and is made of bamboo or wood. Get the largest one you can, so you have ample space to cut your vegetables.
- *Knives.* These are arguably the most useful tools in your kitchen—or at least the most used. A good knife is not only safer, it cuts more evenly. A dull or cheap knife makes cutting a chore, so you're less likely to do it, which means you will be less likely to use the full array of fruits and vegetables you and your family could enjoy. There are three knives every kitchen should have: (1) an eight- to ten-inch chef's knife for chopping herbs and vegetables and slicing meat; (2) a paring knife for more precise cutting, such as slicing strawberries, peeling and coring apples, or deveining shrimp; and (3) a serrated knife for slicing bread.
- *Mandoline slicer.* A great manual tool for slicing vegetables like zucchini and potatoes effortlessly. Always use the guard handle to protect your fingers, or wear a protective glove specifically made for mandolines.
- *Wooden spoons.* Ubiquitous in Blue Zones, these inexpensive, nice-looking, bacteria-resistant implements make cooking easy. Put them in a handsome jar or on the countertop for easy access along with spatulas, slotted spoons, and tongs.
- *Cast-iron pans.* These will last a lifetime if properly cared for and are less expensive than high-end pans. They are naturally nonstick once seasoned and can be superheated to sear meat with minimal oil. They add trace iron to every dish you cook in them.
- *Food mill.* This tool is amazing for crushing cooked vegetables and fruit for soups and sauces. Unlike a blender, a mill forces the food through a sieve, separating out the skins and seeds and resulting in a smooth, good-tasting puree.
- *Potato masher.* Once favored by our grandmothers, the lowly potato masher has gone out of style. Too bad! It makes creamy mashed potatoes with way less cleanup than a standard mixer and it can even help make a quick salsa or spread with cooked or canned beans.

- *Box grater.* Hold this inexpensive, four-sided metal tool with one hand and shred fruits and vegetables along one of its several surfaces, creating coarse slivers or fine pulp.
- *Salad spinner.* This functional bowl or basket is vital for drying lettuce and other leafy greens after washing them.
- *Food processor.* This modern convenience is essential to creating fresh, tasty food. It can chop vegetables in a flash—and save the nutrient-rich juice in the canister, juice that has a tendency to slip onto the counter or even get washed down the drain on a cutting board. It can also make smooth doughs and batter in seconds.
- *Immersion blender.* Sometimes called a "stick blender," this handy tool can puree soups right in the pot—no need to dirty other bowls or drag out a big mixer. Look for an immersion blender with a detachable blade housing; just pop it off for easy cleaning.
- *Sieve or colander.* Keep one within easy reach of the sink to use to drain fruits and vegetables. Colanders that sit in the sink are great.
- *Slow cooker.* Cooking at home saves you money, produces healthier, lower-calorie meals, and builds family bonds. So why don't we do it? Recipes are often complex, requiring cookware we don't have and skills we haven't mastered. And the big reason: We don't have time. The secret solution to easy cooking at home: the slow cooker. Many of the recipes in this book allow you to pour five to ten ingredients into a slow cooker in the morning, turn it on low, and forget about it. By dinnertime, you'll have a healthy Blue Zones meal.

Kitchen Checklist

Whenever we work with people living in the cities where we're doing a Blue Zones makeover, I like to give them a checklist of simple actions that they can keep on hand. Each one is another tiny nudge toward longevity. Here's our Blue Zones kitchen checklist. Take a look and see how many things you already do—and how many you could do in the time to come, to move yourself and your family toward health and longevity.

1. Post a sign with the Four Always & Four to Avoid foods on your refrigerator.

How to do it: Create a simple prominent sign (even a sticky note) to remind you of the 4 Always & 4 to Avoid foods (see pages 186–188). Display it on your refrigerator or kitchen bulletin board.

2. Dedicate the center section of your refrigerator to fruits and vegetables.

How to do it: Get in the habit of keeping your healthy foods front and center in your refrigerator. Placing the healthy options at eye level will encourage you to snack mindfully.

3. Use dinner plates no larger than ten inches.

How to do it: Put away your larger plates and just have ten-inch plates within reach. Eating on smaller plates creates the perception of larger portions and tricks the brain into being satisfied with less food.

4. Drink beverages out of tall, narrow glasses—no more than 2.5 inches in diameter.

How to do it: Stock your kitchen with only narrow, cylinder-shaped glasses. We visually measure our drinks by the height, not width, of the glass. Narrower glasses make us think we are drinking more than we are.

5. Create an out-of-the-way junk food location.

How to do it: Put unhealthy snacks and food out of sight and out of reach, on a top or bottom shelf or inside a drawer or cabinet you don't often open. Label the shelf or drawer "Junk Food." Most junk food is consumed because you see it and it looks good. If you're going to have junk food in your house, hiding it from your line of vision will dramatically decrease consumption.

6. Pre-plate your food.

How to do it: Plate your entire meal and put leftovers away before sitting down at the table. Consider putting a "Dish here, Dine there" reminder on the counter, next to the stove. Research has shown that when people pre-plate their food, they consume less than when they serve at the table, family-style, which encourages multiple servings.

7. Remove the TV, cell phones, and computer from your kitchen and dining room.
How to do it: Get your family to agree that the eating environment is a no-electronics zone. Watching TV, listening to fast-paced music, and using electronics in the kitchen or dining room all promote mindless eating.

8. Put a full fresh fruit bowl in the most prominent place in your kitchen.
How to do it: Fill a bowl with your favorite fruit and display in plain view so that every time you walk through your kitchen, it is the first thing you see. Never put chips or packaged sweets in plain view. Placing healthy options in a convenient, well-lit location makes it more likely those foods will be your first choice.

9. Use hand-operated kitchen tools.
How to do it: Get rid of your electric can opener and use a hand-operated one instead. Get a potato masher, a garlic press, and a whisk rather than using a blender or electric mixer. Try squeezing fruit juice by hand. Manual kitchen tasks encourage hand and arm strengthening.

BLUE ZONE YOUR BEDROOM

Most centenarians go to bed shortly after sunset and wake with daybreak; on average they sleep eight hours a day. In at least three Blue Zones a half-hour nap is a daily ritual—very different from our world. Today, according to Gallup, Americans report an average of 6.8 hours of sleep a day; 14 percent of Americans sleep less than 6 hours. This is not enough.

Sleep is necessary for optimal health and well-being, as research repeatedly shows us. Lack of sleep not only increases one's risk of health problems, including obesity, diabetes, cardiovascular disease, and hypertension, but it can also lead to impaired judgment, risky decision-making, and even decreased attractiveness. Aiming for eight hours of sleep each night is ideal to optimize health and longevity.

The keys to getting a good sleep are a relaxing bedtime routine and a bedroom environment that is a sanctuary for sleep. If you look at bedrooms in the Blue Zones, you won't find computers, TVs, or any other electronics. That includes cell phones, which seem to have become bedside companions for many Americans. Yet the 2011 Sleep in America Poll, conducted by the National Sleep Foundation, found that cell phones were a sleep disturbance. Twenty percent of Generation Yers and 18 percent of Generation Zers polled said that at least a few nights a week they are awakened after they go to bed by a phone call, text message, or email coming into their phones.

Blue Zones bedrooms are cool, quiet, and dark. People don't use alarm clocks. Because they sleep enough, they wake up naturally.

And, I might add, maybe there is another advantage to retiring into a quiet, serene bedroom without distractions. In the Blue Zone of Ikaria, more than 80 percent of people between ages 65 and 100 are still having sex. (No enhancement drugs needed.) Sounds like fun, but sex is also a verified longevity enhancer. A study published in the *British Journal of Medicine* tracked 1,000 45- to 59-year-old Welsh men for ten years. The researchers found that men who experienced frequent orgasms had half the coronary heart disease mortality risk as their less orgasmic counterparts. And a longitudinal study of 1,500 Americans found that for middle-aged married women, frequency of orgasm was moderately protective against mortality risk as well. The lesson: An undistracted bedroom can make a difference.

Bedroom Checklist

The checklist below, developed in collaboration with the Cornell Sleep Lab, takes cues from the Blue Zones and couples them with evidence-based information to help improve your bedroom and sleeping habits.

1. Own a comfortable mattress and comfortable pillows.
How to do it: Make sure that your mattress doesn't sag and that it supports you comfortably as you sleep. Any mattress should be replaced every eight to ten years. When choosing a mattress, spend at least ten minutes lying on it to test it out before buying it. Choose comfortable pillows that support your head without crimping your neck.

2. Set the temperature in your bedroom to 65°F at night.
How to do it: Set your thermostat to 65°F at bedtime. If you have a programmable thermostat, have it automatically adjust to 65°F during sleeping hours. Temperatures below 54°F or above 75°F can actually wake you up at night. If 65°F feels a little colder than you'd like, add an extra blanket.

3. Dim the lights an hour before bed.
How to do it: Try to get into the habit of dimming all the lights in your home an hour before you go to bed. Dimming the lights before bedtime prepares your body for sleep, allowing you to fall asleep faster and stay asleep longer. It's a step toward the darkness you need, explained in the next item in this checklist.

4. Remove digital alarm clocks with lit-up screens.
How to do it: If you can't do without a clock, turn it around so the lit-up screen faces away from the bed while you are sleeping. Research has demonstrated that nighttime light exposure suppresses the production of melatonin, the major hormone secreted by the pineal gland that controls sleep and wake cycles. Even the LED light from digital alarm clocks can suppress melatonin. Hiding your clock from your line of sight will also help you avoid obsessive clock-watching during the night.

5. Use shades, blinds, or drapery to block outside light from coming into your bedroom while you are sleeping.
How to do it: Light, including city streetlights or outdoor security lights, can disrupt sleep. Hang light-blocking window shades or heavy drapery

that can block out all outside light to make your room as dark as possible for the best sleep.

6. Remove the TV, computer, and cell phones from the bedroom.
How to do it: Consider your bedroom a no-electronics zone. By removing the light source and the distraction, you are creating an environment conducive to calm and a deeper, more restful, and healthful sleep.

OTHER WAYS TO BLUE ZONE YOUR HOME

Many simple choices you make about the design of your house and the pathway of your everyday life impact your longevity, in ways you might never have considered. Did you know that watering houseplants burns the same number of calories as stretching and walking, for example? Scientists at the Mayo Clinic found that increasing simple movements such as standing and walking can help you burn an additional 350 calories each day. Another study that examined the lifestyle of San Francisco dockworkers found that those who had regular bursts of activity had lower chances of heart disease.

By deconveniencing your home, or changing the environment to make active living easier, you can burn extra calories without even thinking about it. Preparing food by hand is one way, but there are many others. Don't use items of convenience like a TV remote or a riding lawn mower, for example. By removing these items and adding a little bit of movement all the time to your day, you can seamlessly add physical activity and contribute to your health and longevity.

Helping to put physical activity back into people's lives is one of the most important things we're doing in the 24 American cities where we're re-creating Blue Zones living. We're not going to solve America's obesity epidemic with exercise. The average American only burns 100 calories per day engaged in exercise. The key to losing weight and staying young is to engineer back into our daily lives all the ways we use up calories that modern conveniences have cut out.

Here's a list of common tasks we do around our house and the calories they burn. As you can see, they add up fast. (Calorie counts assume one hour of work by a 190-pound man.)

- Hanging storm windows: 272 calories
- Building a fence: 340 calories
- Laying tile: 238 calories
- Sanding floors: 238 calories
- Spreading dirt with a shovel: 272 calories
- Washing a fence: 238 calories
- Roofing: 340 calories
- Plumbing and wiring: 136 calories
- Shoveling snow: 576 calories
- Raking leaves: 384 calories
- Mowing the lawn: 400 calories

Our grandparents didn't need treadmills to stay in shape, and neither do we. Just do your own chores. You'll not only please your spouse—you'll look and feel better too.

Home and Yard Checklist

Here is a checklist of ways to deconvenience your home to set up your personal living environment with nudges to keep moving all day long. The Mayo Clinic estimates that optimizing your home can burn an extra 150 calories a day. That may not sound like a big deal, but 150 calories a day could add up to six fewer pounds in a year!

1. Place a scale in a prominent spot in your home and weigh yourself daily.
How to do it: Place your scale on the floor in front of your bathroom mirror or in a place where you can't avoid it and get into the habit of using it. Daily weight checks take only seconds, and the results can provide powerful reinforcement. Studies have found that people who

weigh themselves every day weigh less than people who never weigh themselves.

One of our advisers, Robert Jeffery, has spent more than 30 years studying obesity and trying to learn how to prevent it. He says there are very few, if any, universal long-term strategies for fighting weight gain, but one thing that seems to work is self-weighing. Jeffery's team followed 63 individuals for six months and found that people who stepped on the scale weekly lost 7 pounds more than those who weighed themselves less than once a month. And those who stepped on the scale daily lost a whopping 15 pounds during that period. Another study followed more than 2,500 women in the Pacific Northwest for two years and found that women who measured their weight daily weighed 17 pounds less after two years compared with the women who never weighed themselves. It may be that seeing a lower weight on the scales provides positive reinforcement, while seeing a higher weight delivers a gentle kick in the pants to pay attention to what you're eating.

Research shows that the mere act of measuring—whether it's stepping on a scale, taking a health risk assessment, or wearing a step-counter— creates improvement in health. Maybe measuring sets a baseline, helping a person observe and manage better habits. Or maybe measuring makes a person confront just how unhealthy he or she is and prompts that person into action.

Here's one other measurement that can make a big difference for you: the Blue Zones Vitality Compass *(apps.bluezones.com/vitality)*, a simple online longevity assessment tool we developed with Robert L. Kane, an aging specialist, and researchers at the University of Minnesota School of Public Health. It is free to the general public and, with a few short questions, calculates your healthy life expectancy and indicates ways you can improve it. Since we debuted the Vitality Compass in 2008, more than a million people have taken it. We've found that those who take it twice report behaviors that yield an extra 1.6 years of life expectancy. We suspect that the Vitality Compass, by just making people aware of what and how much certain behaviors contributes to longevity, prompts positive behavior change.

2. Have only one TV in your home.

How to do it: Put your television in a common room, preferably in a cabinet behind doors. The goal here is to nudge you away from mindless screen time that encourages overeating and detracts from potential physical activity. In short, people who watch too much TV are more likely to be overweight. Watching TV actually lowers the metabolism. We become less active and engaged, and we're more inclined to eat junk food. Kids with a TV in their bedroom are 18 percent more likely to be (or become) obese—and to have lower grades in school. Centenarians in the Blue Zones don't even watch television, and the happiest people in North America watch only 30 to 60 minutes of television per day.

3. Replace power tools with hand tools.

How to do it: Mow your lawn with a push lawn mower, shovel the snow with a hand shovel, and gather the leaves from your lawn with an old-fashioned rake. Shoveling, raking, and push-mowing are healthy and productive outdoor workouts—some burn almost 400 calories an hour. In fact, mowing the lawn or raking leaves burns about the same amount of calories as lifting weights. And it gets the chores done at the same time.

4. Grow and maintain your own garden.

How to do it: If you have a yard, designate a spot for a garden. Plant a garden, and for the next four to six months, you're coaxed every day to water, weed, hoe, prune, and harvest. Gardening is exactly the type of low-intensity, range-of-motion, easy-on-the-joints physical activity that is sustainable for the long run. You can burn 150 calories by gardening (standing) for approximately 30 to 45 minutes. Also, research shows that gardening lowers stress hormones.

In most Blue Zones, the kitchen garden is an extension of the food preparation area. Nicoyans traditionally cook in outdoor kitchens set among a garden grove of papaya, citrus, and other tropical fruits. In Okinawa, right outside the back door grew green onions, turmeric, mugwort, and garlic—always fresh and always accessible. We forget that fresh fruits, vegetables, and herbs begin to degrade, or oxidize, as soon as we pick them. A fresh source at hand ensures quality in the food we eat.

5. Own a dog.

How to do it: Go to your local animal shelter to adopt or to a pet store to buy a dog. Pets make great companions, and dogs especially encourage you to walk or run regularly. Researchers found that if you own a dog, you get over five hours of exercise a week without a lot of added effort.

6. Add bicycle riding to your routines.

How to do it: Buy a bike and helmet if you don't already have them. Fix your current bike if you do. Just having a functioning bike nudges you to use it. Riding a bicycle at a moderate speed burns approximately 235 calories per half hour. And the helmet is important for longevity too: Wearing a bicycle helmet reduces the risk of serious head injury in crashes by as much as 85 percent and the risk of brain injury by as much as 88 percent.

7. Take up your favorite sports, including running and camping.

How to do it: I encourage people living in the cities doing Blue Zones makeovers to be sure they own at least four of the following: basketball, baseball, football, golf balls and clubs, in-line skates, camping supplies, running shoes. And to use them for fun and pleasure! Did you know that in-line skating burns more calories than running track and field hurdles, and that playing catch for only 30 minutes burns more than 100 calories? Keep your sporting equipment in good condition and close at hand, easy to find and easy to use.

8. Grow indoor plants throughout your home.

How to do it: Pick up some pots, potting soil, and some of your favorite greenery to place throughout your home. For plants that are easy to maintain, try a golden pothos vine or a spider plant. Watering plants around the house burns the same amount of calories as stretching and walking. Besides their ability to clean the air, indoor plants have been proven to provide health benefits to people who interact with them. And because plants are in your home, along your everyday pathway, you'll be nudged to nurture them regularly.

9. Create a destination room.

How to do it: Designate a room on the top level of your home as your family's Blue Zones destination. Include a large table for family projects, shelves filled with books, and plenty of light. Leave out the clock, TV, computer, or other distracting gadgets. It's a place where anyone in your family can go to be fully immersed in what he or she is doing—engage in a hobby, read a book, or do a family activity. Why upstairs? Because a popular room on another level of your home increases stair climbing, and even doing that will increase the physical activity in your daily life. You burn ten calories per minute climbing up stairs and four calories per minute climbing down them.

10. Disconnect your garage door opener.

How to do it: Stop using your electric garage door opener. Instead, open the door manually. Getting out of the car, raising the door, and returning to the car rather than using a remote control will burn seven calories per minute. Doing this twice a day takes about 10 minutes and burns around 70 additional calories!

11. Create an indoor exercise area.

How to do it: Reserve part of a room in your home for exercise equipment, a stability ball, a yoga mat, or a weight set. If exercising is more convenient, you're more likely to do it. A study at the University of Florida found that women who exercised at home lost 25 pounds in 15 months and maintained that loss.

12. Get rid of your TV remote control.

How to do it: Instead of using a remote control to change the channel or operate the DVD player, walk over to your equipment and do it manually. Changing the channel manually will burn ten calories every time you get up.

13. Optimize your furniture.

How to do it: Instead of sitting on chairs and furniture all the time, sit on cushions on the floor. You will work your thighs, glutes, and lower back each time you sit down and stand back up, and you'll also be supporting yourself without a chair back, which improves your posture and can burn up to an additional 130 calories each hour. Also, install a stand-up desk for paper/computer work at home. Standing instead of sitting at a desk can burn an extra 300 calories per day.

YOUR *MOAI*—CREATING YOUR OWN BLUE ZONE BY CURATING A CIRCLE OF FRIENDS

As I have found through all my journeys to the Blue Zones of the world, one of the most dependable, universal means to greater health and happiness is to simply socialize more. In fact, according to the Robert Wood Johnson Foundation, loneliness can be as bad for you as a smoking habit, shaving years off your life expectancy. Data from Gallup-Healthways polls on well-being show that the happiest people socialize at least eight hours a day—especially with their parents and family. An analysis by Nicholas Christakis, a social scientist at Harvard and one of our Blue Zones Project advisers, showed that in a network of more than 5,000 people living in a small Massachusetts town, the happiest people were also the most connected. As their social circle got happier, so did they. Even introverts are happier around people than when they're alone, studies have shown. So for the vast majority of us, setting up our lives to make it easier to socialize will increase both health and happiness.

The quantity of social interaction is only half of the prescription. Quality matters too. The sort of people we hang out with has an enormous and measurable influence not only on how happy we are, but also on how fat or even how lonely we are. On any given Tuesday night, we can sit in a bar and listen to an old acquaintance's problems—or we can spend that evening going to the theater with an upbeat friend. According to one statistical analysis, each additional happy friend we have in our social circle boosts our cheeriness by 9 percent, while each additional unhappy friend drags it down by 7 percent. Similarly, if your three best friends are obese, there's a 55 percent better chance that you'll be overweight yourself. Since friends are long-term adventures, surrounding ourselves with the right people, and engineering our lives so we spend more time with those people, is going to have a profound, long-term impact on our happiness and longevity.

In fact, just being around happy people will impact our well-being. Behaviors, it seems, spread partly through subconscious social signals—so-called "mirror neurons"—that we pick up from those around us. For example, we tend to automatically mimic what we see in the faces of those around us, which is why looking at a photograph of smiling people can itself often lift your mood. So just hanging out in a café with upbeat people can add a bit of happiness to your day.

In Blue Zones, people don't go on diets, work out at gyms, or take supplements. Instead, they surround themselves with the right kinds of friends. In Okinawa people keep a *moai,* a group of friends, for a lifetime. When things go well—they have a good crop, they get a raise—they are expected to share the benefits. Conversely, when things go south—a parent dies, they get divorced, or they experience inevitable frailty—they can always count on their moai for real and psychological support. (Maybe that's why Okinawan women are the world's longest-lived population.)

We now know that health behaviors are as contagious as catching a cold.

Here are some ideas on how to be sure you are part of a social circle with the greatest longevity benefits.

Social Circle Checklist

1. Assess your current circle of friends.
How to do it: Using all the ideas in this book about the healthy lifestyles of people living to 100 in the Blue Zones, take a look at the people who form your social world right now. Here is a list of questions we developed in collaboration with the University of Minnesota School of Public Health that will help you determine if your friends are having a

positive or negative influence on your health. While we wouldn't tell you to drop your old friends, we might encourage you to spend more time with your positive friends or augment your circle of friends to include more positive influences.

- Do they smoke?
- Are they overweight because of bad health behavior?
- Do they drink more than two drinks a day?
- Do they eat a mostly plant-based diet?
- Do they cook at home?
- Do they favor junk food or whole food?
- Are they usually upbeat or do they like to complain?
- Is their idea of recreation watching TV or an outdoor activity?
- Are they curious about the world?
- Do they listen as well as talk?
- Are they engaged with the world and encourage your engagement?
- Are they tied to routine or interested in new activities?
- Do you feel better around them than when you're not?

You get the idea here. Research shows we start mimicking the behavior and even the feelings of our close friends. So while I won't necessarily tell you to dump your old, toxic friends, I will tell you that you'll set yourself up for better health behaviors long term if you carefully cultivate your closest social circle.

2. Join a club.

How to do it: Think about what your interests or talents are and find an organization that will nurture them. The idea here is to make a commitment to some club, volunteer group, or social organization—a sphere of people with common interests that compels you to show up regularly, either because of organizational rules or out of peer pressure (if not simply out of the pleasure you gain from the associations). According to one study, joining a group that meets even once a month produces the same happiness gain as doubling your income.

3. Create your own moai.

How to do it: Be the glue that brings together a group of mutually committed friends, reminiscent of an Okinawan moai. Okinawans, the world's longest-lived people, travel through life together in clusters of five friends, as described in chapter 2. They commit to meeting regularly, share spoils in the case of a windfall, and support each other in times of crisis or grief. In our Blue Zones Project cities we create these moais. To work, the moai participants need to be ready to change, need to live near one another, and need to reflect on one another's health initiatives—three unspoken rules that derive from widely accepted social theories.

So whenever we enter a community that wants to transform itself, we build moais by inviting people who are ready to do three things: change their health habits, meet people like themselves, and spread the health epidemic. At the initial meeting to organize moais, we first break up the group into circles of 20 to 50 people. A facilitator throws out questions that get people thinking about what they like: "Raise your hand if you've watched a Disney movie in the last three months," or "Raise your hand if you've been to church in the past month," or "Raise your hand if you've been to a bar in the last week." Participants are instructed to note others they might like to get to know.

After a couple dozen questions, we ask people to organize themselves into groups of five or six people with shared interests, such as new mothers, or those who like sports, or those who tend to volunteer. Then for the next ten weeks those groups get together to walk, enough times so people really get to know their moai members. They might also host potluck dinners based on Blue Zones food guidelines. We found that in Albert Lea, Minnesota, a full 60 percent of people who joined moais were still members three years later!

4. Join a church.

How to do it: Just about every study done on the connection between religion and longevity shows that the two go hand in hand. While we're not sure if churchgoing makes you live long or living longer makes you want to go to church, research shows that people who belong to a faith-based community and attend at least four times per month live four to fourteen years longer than people who don't (and it doesn't matter if they're Christian, Muslim, Buddhist, Hindu, or Jewish). Churchgoers are less likely to engage in risky behaviors, are satisfied with less money, experience less stress, and have built-in social networks. And research shows you'll amplify the longevity benefits of belonging to a faith community if you become active: join the choir, volunteer as a greeter, or commit to read for the congregation. If you don't belong, or have drifted away from the faith community of your birth, try to find a new one that matches your current values and worldview. Start by asking friends or people you admire to make some suggestions. If you are not sure, attend service in a different location once a week for the next eight weeks.

THE BIG PICTURE

Most of us spend about 80 percent of our lives within about a 20-mile radius of our homes. We have direct control over how we set up our kitchen, bedroom, yard, and even social network, but managing our bigger life radius is more difficult. Do you live in a community where sodas, salty snacks, and fast food are the cheapest and most accessible choices, or one where subsidies and tax policy favor fruits and vegetables? Are parks maintained? Can you take a bus to work, and can your kids walk to school, or does every trip require you to get into your car? Do zoning ordinances encourage sprawl or favor a vibrant, active inner-city core? What I have found by working with communities eager to make big changes toward health and longevity is that these sorts of things make an even bigger difference than an individual person's diet or exercise program.

Although you may not realize it, you have the power to improve some aspects of your life radius. In our Blue Zones Project communities, I've seen people join food action committees to introduce public vegetable gardens or propose ordinances to limit the number of fast-food restaurants per block. I've seen people lobby a city council to deny a permit for a convenience store next to the junior high. It sounds like a cliché, but a call or an email to the mayor's office really does work. Your vote helps determine your community leaders. Are they ones who want to build a town for just cars and commerce or ones who build to favor humans and quality of life? Do they perpetuate the convenience trap of more strip malls and highways or advocate for parks and places for people to connect?

The secret to longevity—whether for individuals or communities—does not rest with the federal government. Nor does it rest with the medical community: Doctors aren't going to fix our country's biggest health problems. They're better at making sick people less sick than they are at preventing sickness in the first place. And pharmaceutical companies aren't going to help much: They're primarily in the business of selling drugs to sick people.

The answer—at least for now—lies with the people in your community: the municipal government officials, the people who own the places where you eat and buy food, the school administrators, the large employers, and the mothers and fathers who run households and make daily lifestyle decisions. These are the people who control our living environment from the time we wake up to the time we go to bed. If we arm these people with strategies to nudge us into better eating, more natural movement, and better social interaction, better health will ensue, with longevity an added bonus. It's not a silver bullet, it's silver buckshot: a healthy swarm of small things that add up to a huge impact.

The key to longevity is re-creating the Blue Zones in our lives.

IS IT WORKING?

I recently phoned Bob Fagen at his home in Spencer, Iowa. As you may recall, Bob is the city manager who'd faced an alarming problem he was having with his kidneys and made a difference by adopting Blue Zones behaviors. It was a warm July evening when we spoke, and Bob had just walked home from City Hall, a journey that took him about a mile through leafy neighborhoods and along the footpaths flanking the Sioux River.

Since the Blue Zones Project came to his town, he told me, he's seen the number of people with serious chronic diseases in Spencer drop by 60 percent. Health care costs for city workers had dropped every year, in some cases by 50 percent in a single year. Personally, he's lost more than 50 pounds, he added, and his kidneys are healthy. I asked him if he thought it would all last.

"Well," he said after a pause, "I see all the community gardens that we didn't have before. Watering, weeding. I stop by and talk to the people there, take time I didn't used to take before." He paused and started up again: "I also see a lot more people out walking since the sidewalks went in. People are eating at outdoor restaurants. I see a lot more networking than I did three years ago.

"This Blue Zones thing is a journey," he continued. "Around here, our habits were solidified when we were kids. We used to just put food in our mouths and not really think about it. So the idea that we should be eating vegetables felt like a challenge until we tried them and discovered we actually liked them. Now my grandkids are learning the healthy habits from my daughter from the get-go—not just eating vegetables, but eating at the supper table instead of eating on the run like I did."

"But how about you personally, Bob?" I pressed. "How have you changed?"

"Put it this way," he finally answered. "I live in the 'pork state,' and now I actually sort of think kale is cool."

PART FOUR

Blue Zones
Recipes

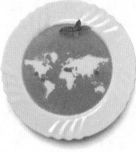

77 Easy, Delicious Recipes

NOW THE FUN PART! Here are some of my favorite recipes, both those that come from my friends who live in the Blue Zones and those that I have found here at home that work well in a Blue Zones food plan. Some of the recipes are 100 percent traditional, and some have been adapted for American kitchens, using ingredients that are readily available in any supermarket.

Remember, when it comes to longevity, there's no short-term fix. So try these foods and recipes until you find which ones you like the best, so you will keep on eating them for a long time—all the way to 100.

BEAN-BASED RECIPES

LENTIL SOUP

<u>Yield: 6 servings</u>

Lentils are popular in all cultures where a lot of beans are eaten because they are so simple to prepare. They need no soaking and they cook up in no time. They're inexpensive and available year-round. Although they come in green, brown, red, or black varieties, skip the red lentils for this easy soup; they'll just dissolve into mush. Instead, use either green (sometimes called French lentils or lentils du Puy), brown, or black lentils; the green or black ones will hold their shape and texture better to make a brothier, lighter meal; the brown ones will break down a bit and give the soup a richer, thicker consistency. It's your call for your preference.

½ pound (1¼ cups) green, black, or brown lentils
7 cups (1 quart plus 3 cups) vegetable broth
2 large red globe, beefsteak, or heirloom tomatoes, chopped (about 1½ cups)
1 medium yellow or white onion, chopped (about 1 cup)
2 medium carrots, peeled and chopped (about ⅔ cup)
2 medium red potatoes, peeled and chopped (about ⅔ cup)
2 bay leaves
½ teaspoon salt
Finely chopped scallions, for garnish
Extra-virgin olive oil, for garnish

1. Spread the lentils on a large baking sheet and pick them over for any bits of stone.
2. Stir the lentils, broth, tomatoes, onion, carrots, potatoes, bay leaves, and salt in a large saucepan or soup pot. Bring to a simmer over medium-high heat. Reduce the heat to low, set a lid askew over the pan or pot, and cook until the lentils are soft, for 45 minutes.
3. Discard the bay leaves. Ladle the soup into bowls. Garnish each with scallions and up to 1 teaspoon olive oil.

Tip: For extra flavor, cook the chopped onion and carrot in 1 tablespoon olive oil for 5 to 7 minutes in the saucepan or soup pot set over medium heat before adding the remainder of the ingredients indicated in step 1.

Tip: Change the recipe a little by adding up to 1 cup packed baby spinach, baby kale, baby arugula, stemmed watercress, or a mixture of any to the soup after it has simmered for 35 minutes. Continue cooking with the lid askew for 10 minutes, until the lentils are tender and the greens have wilted.

Tip: For an easier prep, use frozen chopped onion (no need to thaw).

🍴 SPICED LENTILS

<u>Yield: 4 servings</u>

This recipe makes a great main course, sort of like a well-dressed, warm lentil salad. Eat it alongside Horta (page 246) or a tossed green salad.

1½ cups green lentils (also called French lentils or lentils *du Puy*) or black beluga
    lentils
2 tablespoons extra-virgin olive oil or canola oil
1 large yellow or white onion, chopped (about 1½ cups)
1½ tablespoons fresh lemon juice
1 tablespoon minced peeled fresh ginger
½ teaspoon chili powder
½ teaspoon mild paprika
½ teaspoon salt

1. Spread the lentils on a large baking sheet and pick them over for small stones.
2. Place the lentils in a medium saucepan and add enough water so they're submerged by 2 inches. Bring to a simmer over high heat; then reduce the heat to low and cook, uncovered, until tender, about 25 minutes. Drain in a colander set over a bowl, reserving the cooking water below.
3. Warm the oil in a large skillet set over medium heat. Add the onion and cook, stirring often, until softened, about 5 minutes. Stir in the lentils, lemon juice, ginger, chili powder, paprika, and salt. Stir until fragrant, about 1 minute. If the dish seems too dry, add the reserved cooking liquid in 2-tablespoon increments until a bit saucy without being soupy. Serve warm.

Tip: If desired, cover the completed recipe in the skillet and set in a 250°F oven for up to 1 hour, until you're ready to eat. Check occasionally and stir in more of the reserved cooking liquid if the dish seems too dry.

🍴 BASIC COOKED BEANS

Yield: 6 cups cooked beans

Beans are a top Blue Zones protein, so there are a lot of bean recipes in this book. Canned beans are a shortcut, but dried beans save you big time on money and sodium. Using them also keeps more of the beans' nutrients intact. Preparing dried beans in advance is easy with a slow cooker. Make a large batch of beans and divide it into meal-size servings to freeze for later.

1 pound dried pinto, black, red kidney, great northern, cannellini, or cranberry beans
1 large yellow or white onion, chopped (about 1½ cups)
1 tablespoon minced garlic
1 teaspoon dried thyme
½ teaspoon salt

1. Spread the beans on a large baking sheet and discard any that are discolored or broken. Set the beans in a large bowl and add enough cool tap water so they're submerged by 2 inches. Soak at room temperature for at least 8 hours but no more than 16 hours (that is, overnight).
2. Drain the beans in a colander set in the sink. Pour them into a 4- to 6-quart slow cooker; add the onion, garlic, and thyme. Stir in 5 cups water.
3. Cover and cook until the beans are tender, about 5 hours on high or 9 to 10 hours on low.
4. Stir in the salt, cover, and cook for 10 more minutes. Uncover and let the beans cool, storing them with their cooking liquid in small, sealed containers in the refrigerator for up to 4 days or in the freezer for up to 4 months.

Tip: Red kidney beans can cause a particularly nasty stomach upset in a small percentage of the population. Solve this by boiling the soaked and drained beans in a large saucepan of water for 5 minutes before draining and adding to the slow cooker. Never cook red kidney beans in their soaking water (in fact, you increase the chance of *minor* stomach upset by cooking any dried bean in its soaking water).

Tip: If you don't want to soak the beans overnight, set them in a large saucepan and add enough cool water so they're submerged by 2 inches; bring to a full, rolling boil over high heat, stirring occasionally. Remove from the heat, cover, and set aside for 1 hour. Continue with step 2 of the recipe.

¶¶ BLACK BEAN SOUP

Yield: 4 servings

This variation on a dish found in many of the Blue Zones adds fruit and spices for intense flavor. Don't be put off by the long list of ingredients; most of them are spices, so the recipe is easy and fast! A green salad and some corn tortillas or sourdough rolls alongside it will make a meal.

2 tablespoons extra-virgin olive oil
1 medium yellow or white onion, diced (about 1 cup)
4 medium celery ribs, diced (about 1 cup)
½ medium red bell pepper, cored, seeded, and diced (about ⅓ cup)
1 large red globe, beefsteak, or heirloom tomato, chopped (about ¾ cup)
1 tablespoon minced garlic
3½ cups cooked black beans plus 2 cups cooking liquid
2 cups vegetable broth
1 tablespoon finely grated orange zest

1 teaspoon ground cumin
1 teaspoon dried oregano
1½ teaspoons celery seeds
½ teaspoon ground allspice
½ teaspoon ground cloves
½ teaspoon ground cinnamon
½ teaspoon salt
1 medium pineapple, peeled, cored, and cut into 1-inch-thick rings (optional)

1. Warm the oil in a large soup pot or Dutch oven set over medium heat. Add the onion, celery, and bell pepper; cook, stirring often, until softened, about 8 minutes.
2. Add the tomato and garlic; cook, stirring occasionally, until the tomatoes begin to break down, about 5 minutes.
3. Add the beans with their liquid or water, broth, zest, all the spices, and the salt. Increase the heat to high and bring to a full simmer, stirring occasionally. Cover, reduce the heat to low, and simmer slowly until slightly thickened and mellowed in its flavors, about 30 minutes.
4. If desired, grill the pineapple slices in a nonstick grill pan set over medium-high heat, turning once, until marked and tender, about 6 minutes; or broil on a large, lipped baking sheet 4 to 6 inches from a heated broiler for 4 minutes, turning once. Cut into chunks. Serve the soup with the pineapple on top or on the side.

Tip: If you do not have precooked black beans, use 2 (15-ounce) cans black beans, drained and rinsed (about 3½ cups) and increase the vegetable broth to 4 cups (1 quart).

Tip: When the soup is finished, partially blend with an immersion blender, if you want a thicker soup with a few chunky bits in it.

¶¶ SPICY BEAN BURGERS

Yield: 4 burgers

I love vegetarian burgers, but the ones I find frozen in the supermarket leave me lukewarm. You have to load those up with a lot of vegetables to disguise the taste! That's why I love this recipe. The burgers themselves are tasty, and I can then use the vegetables to enhance their flavor rather than disguise it. If you like your burgers less spicy, use less red pepper sauce.

4 cups cooked and drained pinto beans or drained and rinsed canned pinto beans
¾ cup fresh whole-grain bread crumbs

Up to 1 tablespoon bottled hot red pepper sauce, such as Tabasco

2 teaspoons minced garlic

½ tablespoon Salsa Lizano (see page 291) or Worcestershire sauce

½ teaspoon ground cumin

½ teaspoon salt

Nonstick spray

4 whole-grain hamburger buns

½ cup Avocado Salsa (page 284) or *pico de gallo*

4 small Romaine lettuce leaves

4 green bell pepper slices (optional)

4 thin red onion rings (optional)

1. Put the beans, bread crumbs, hot red pepper sauce, garlic, Salsa Lizano or Worcestershire sauce, cumin, and salt in a large bowl. Use a potato masher to blend these ingredients into a smooth paste. Cover and refrigerate for 30 minutes to firm up.

2. Spray the grate of an outdoor gas grill with nonstick spray, cover, and heat to high. Or spray a large grill pan with nonstick spray and set over medium-high heat for a few minutes until hot.

3. Meanwhile, use clean, wet hands to form the bean mixture into four even patties, each about 5 inches in diameter and ½-inch thick. Grill the patties until hot and a little crisp, about 6 minutes, turning once.

4. Place the patties on the bottom of the buns and top each with 2 tablespoons Avocado Salsa or pico de gallo, as well as the lettuce and the tops of those buns. Garnish with pepper slices and onion rings as desired.

Tip: You can also make these burgers with a combination of pinto and black beans.

Tip: As long as you've got the grill or the grill pan hot, toast the buns cut side down for less than 1 minute, until marked and lightly browned.

¶¶ SLOW-COOKED VEGETARIAN BLACK BEAN AND POTATO STEW

Yield: 6 servings

If you like heat, use hot chili powder or even pure ancho chili powder. If you like a milder soup, use less—or even none and substitute with mild paprika or even sweet smoked paprika.

1 (28-ounce) can crushed tomatoes, preferably fire-roasted tomatoes (about 3½ cups)

3 cups cooked black beans without their cooking liquid or drained and rinsed canned black beans

2 cups vegetable broth

2 medium sweet potatoes (about 1¼ pounds total weight), peeled and cut into cubes

1 cup cooked and drained red kidney beans or drained and rinsed canned red kidney beans

1 medium yellow or white onion, chopped (about 1 cup)

2 medium red potatoes (about 12 ounces total weight), cut into cubes

2 tablespoons minced garlic

2 teaspoons chili powder

1 teaspoon ground cumin

½ teaspoon salt

1 cored and diced red bell pepper, for garnish

Finely chopped scallions, for garnish

Finely chopped fresh cilantro leaves, for garnish

1. Stir the tomatoes, black beans, broth, sweet potatoes, kidney beans, onion, red potatoes, garlic, chili powder, cumin, and salt in a 5- to 6-quart slow cooker. Cover and cook on high for 4 hours or on low for 8 hours.
2. Ladle into bowls and garnish with bell pepper, scallions, and cilantro.

¶¶ WHITE BEAN AND ROOT VEGETABLE CASSEROLE

Yield: 6 servings

This vegetarian main course is comfort food for a cold winter night. Save back the leftovers in a sealed container in the fridge for up to 2 days or in the freezer for up to 4 months.

2 tablespoons extra-virgin olive oil

1 medium yellow or white onion, chopped (about 1 cup)

1 tablespoon minced garlic

1 (28-ounce) can diced tomatoes, preferably fire-roasted tomatoes (about 3½ cups)

2 cups cooked and drained great northern beans or drained and rinsed canned great northern beans

2 cups cooked and drained cannellini beans or drained and rinsed canned cannellini beans

2 large carrots, peeled and cut into ½-inch chunks

1 large turnip (about 6 ounces), peeled and cut into ½-inch cubes

1 large parsnip (about 4 ounces), peeled and cut into ½-inch chunks

½ cup vegetable broth

1 teaspoon dried oregano
Up to 1 teaspoon ground dried cayenne
½ teaspoon salt
1 cup fresh whole-grain bread crumbs
3 tablespoons chopped fresh parsley leaves

1. Position the rack in the lower third of the oven and heat the oven to 400°F.
2. Warm 1 tablespoon of the oil in a large oven-safe Dutch oven or cast-iron oval casserole set over medium heat. Add the onion and cook, stirring often, until softened, about 5 minutes. Add the garlic and stir until aromatic, about 20 seconds.
3. Stir in the tomatoes, both beans, carrots, turnip, parsnip, broth, oregano, cayenne, and salt. Raise the heat to high and bring to a full simmer. Cover and place in the oven. Bake for 40 minutes.
4. Meanwhile, warm the remaining 1 tablespoon of oil in a small skillet set over medium heat. Add the bread crumbs and parsley. Stir until coated. Set aside off the heat.
5. Uncover the pot or casserole and spread the bread crumb mixture evenly on top of the vegetables. Bake, uncovered, for 20 more minutes, or until the bread crumbs are toasted and the vegetables are tender. Cool for 5 minutes before serving in bowls.

Tip: If you don't care for parsnips, use a small sweet potato, peeled and diced.

¶ BLUE ZONES PORK AND BEANS

Yield: 6 servings

Pork and beans is almost as American as apple pie and, yes, it fits into a Blue Zones diet as a celebratory food because of the small amount of pork that's used as a flavoring. I like to flavor it with a dark beer but almost any kind will do (just no chocolate stouts or raspberry wheats).

1 tablespoon extra-virgin olive oil
2 medium yellow or white onions, chopped (about 2 cups)
Up to 1 small jalapeño, stemmed, cored, and minced
1 tablespoon minced garlic
12 ounces center-cut boneless pork loin chops, finely diced
2½ cups cooked and drained pinto beans or drained and rinsed canned pinto beans
1 (14-ounce) can diced tomatoes, preferably fire-roasted tomatoes (about 1¾ cups)
1 (12-ounce) bottle dark beer (about 1½ cups), such as porter

½ teaspoon salt
½ teaspoon freshly ground black pepper
Finely chopped fresh cilantro leaves, for garnish
Lime wedges, for garnish

1. Warm the oil in a large saucepan or Dutch oven set over medium heat. Add the onions and cook, stirring often, until softened, about 7 minutes. Add the jalapeño and garlic; cook until aromatic, about 1 minute.
2. Add the pork and cook, stirring occasionally, until no longer pink, about 7 minutes. Stir in the beans, tomatoes, beer, salt, and pepper. Raise the heat to medium-high and bring to a boil.
3. Reduce the heat to low and simmer slowly, uncovered, until somewhat thickened, about 10 minutes. Serve in bowls, sprinkled with cilantro as a garnish. Also, offer lime wedges to squeeze over each helping and brighten the flavors.

ᵼᵼ INDIAN CHICKPEAS

Yield: 6 servings

Inspired by Indian fare, this dish features healthful chickpeas seasoned with popular Blue Zones spices.

1½ cups dried chickpeas
¼ cup extra-virgin olive oil or canola oil
2 medium yellow or white onions, halved and sliced into thin half-moons
1 tablespoon minced peeled fresh ginger
½ tablespoon ground dried turmeric
½ teaspoon chili powder
2 large red globe, beefsteak, or heirloom tomatoes, chopped (about 1½ cups)
6 fresh mint leaves, torn up
½ teaspoon salt
½ teaspoon freshly ground black pepper
Vegetable broth, as needed
3 tablespoons fresh lemon juice

1. Set the chickpeas in a large bowl, cover with water, and soak for at least 8 hours or up to 16 hours (that is, overnight). Drain in a colander set in the sink, then pour into a large saucepan. Add enough water so they're submerged by 2 inches, then bring to a boil over high heat. Cover and reduce the heat to medium-low. Simmer until tender, about 15 minutes. Drain again in that colander.

2. Warm the oil in a large pot or Dutch oven set over medium heat. Add the onions and cook, stirring often, until limp but not brown, about 5 minutes. Stir in the ginger, turmeric, and chili powder until fragrant, about 20 seconds. Stir in the drained chickpeas, tomatoes, mint leaves, salt, and pepper.
3. Bring to a simmer; then reduce the heat to medium-low and cook, stirring often, until the tomatoes have broken down into a sauce, about 12 minutes. If the mixture begins to dry out, add vegetable broth in 2-tablespoon increments to keep it moist. Stir in the lemon juice and serve.

Tip: Skip soaking and cooking the chickpeas; substitute 2 (15-ounce) cans, drained and rinsed. Add these chickpeas at the end of step 2.

¶ BRENDA'S MAPLE-GINGER RED BEANS

Yield: 4 to 6 servings

Brenda Langton had been cooking Blue Zones foods 30 years before I found the first Blue Zone. Her Minneapolis restaurant, Spoonriver, is my go-to lunch haunt— one of those few restaurants where you can't get an unhealthy or so-so meal. Everything tastes fantastic! As for this recipe we've adapted from The Spoonriver Cookbook: *Better than any baked beans, these red beans are sweet and savory.*

1 cup dried small red beans
½ cup vegetable broth
2 tablespoons maple syrup
2 tablespoons grated fresh ginger
1 tablespoon soy sauce
½ teaspoon salt

1. Soak dried beans in a large bowl of water at room temperature for at least 8 hours or up to 12 hours. Drain and rinse the beans in a colander set in the sink.
2. Put the beans and 3 cups of water in a large pot. Cover and bring to a boil over high heat. Reduce the heat to low and simmer until tender, about 1 hour. Drain in that colander.
3. Return the beans to the pot; set it over medium heat. Stir in the broth, maple syrup, ginger, soy sauce, and salt. Bring to a simmer and cook, stirring frequently, for a couple of minutes longer until slightly thickened before serving.

Tip: Use small red beans, not red kidney beans.

Tip: If you want to add some diced carrots, onions, and celery, cook ½ cup of each in a tablespoon olive oil in a large skillet over medium heat for 5 minutes, stirring often, then add to the beans with the broth.

Tip: You can also use 2½ cups drained and rinsed canned beans or precooked beans; simply skip steps 1 and 2 and add them in step 3 with the other ingredients.

🍴 LIA'S BLACK BEANS

Yield: 4 servings

Sometimes you don't have time to fix dried beans from scratch. My friend Lia Miller, who researches many of the best recipes at the New York Times, *has the secret to making black beans from the can seem "done from scratch." Try the same approach with other canned beans.*

¼ cup diced yellow or white onion
2 garlic cloves, finely minced
1 tablespoon extra-virgin olive oil, or more as necessary
1 (15-ounce) can black beans, drained and rinsed
½ teaspoon ground cumin
½ teaspoon dried oregano
¼ teaspoon ground bay leaf
Salt and pepper
2 tablespoons Herdez salsa casera or other spicy salsa

1. Cook the onion and garlic in olive oil in a medium saucepan over medium heat, stirring often, until soft but not browned, about 4 minutes. Stir in the beans.
2. Cook until heated through, 3 to 5 minutes. Don't let the beans stick; add a tablespoon or so of water or a little more olive oil if necessary.
4. Take a masher or back of spoon and mush some of the beans.
5. Stir in the cumin, oregano, bay leaf, salt and pepper to taste.
6. At the last minute, add the Herdez salsa casera or other spicy salsa.

🍴 MICHELE SCICOLONE'S GIANT BEANS IN TOMATO SAUCE

Yield: 8 servings

Michele Scicolone has written widely about Italian and Mediterranean cooking, including many, many cookbooks. This tasty recipe comes from her 2013 book The Mediterranean Slow Cooker.

1 pound dried gigantes or large lima beans, rinsed, drained, and picked over
2 tablespoons extra-virgin olive oil

2 large yellow or white onions, chopped (about 3 cups)
2 medium celery ribs, chopped (about ½ cup)
2 medium carrots, peeled and chopped (about ⅔ cup)
3 large garlic cloves, finely chopped
¼ cup tomato paste
Salt and freshly ground pepper
7 cups water
Pinch red pepper flakes
1 bay leaf
1 teaspoon dried oregano
½ teaspoon dried thyme
1 cup crumbled feta cheese (about 8 ounces)
¼ cup finely chopped fresh Italian flat-leaf parsley leaves

1. Place the beans to soak in a large bowl with cold water to cover by several inches. Let stand at room temperature for 6 hours or in the refrigerator overnight.
2. In a large skillet, heat the oil over medium heat. Add the onions, celery, and carrots. Cook, stirring occasionally, until tender, about 10 minutes. Stir in the garlic and cook for 1 minute. Add the tomato paste, 1 teaspoon salt, and pepper to taste.
3. Add the water, red pepper flakes, bay leaf, oregano, and thyme. Bring the mixture to a simmer. Pour it into a large slow cooker.
4. Drain the beans and place them in the slow cooker. Cover and cook on low for 6 to 8 hours, or until the beans are very tender. Taste for seasonings.
5. Just before serving, discard the bay leaf. If there is too much liquid, mash some of the beans into the sauce. Stir in the cheese. Sprinkle with the parsley and serve hot.

🍴 MARK BITTMAN'S STEWED CHICKPEAS WITH CHICKEN

Yield: 6 servings

This Mark Bittman dish features one of the favorite beans of Sardinia and Ikaria—chickpeas—but has seasonings drawn from North Africa. The recipe has been adapted just a bit to fit the smaller amount of meat typical of Blue Zones centenarian eating patterns.

4 cups cooked or drained and rinsed canned chickpeas
2 cups bean-cooking liquid, vegetable stock, or water
Salt and freshly ground black pepper
1 tablespoon neutral oil, like grapeseed or canola

6 chicken legs, skin removed
1 large yellow or white onion, chopped (about 1½ cups)
1 medium celery stalk, chopped (about ¼ cup)
1 medium carrot, peeled and chopped (about ⅓ cup)
1 tablespoon minced garlic
1 teaspoon minced fresh ginger
1 teaspoon ground coriander
2 teaspoons ground cumin
2 cups peeled, seeded, and chopped tomato (canned is fine; include the juices)
Chopped fresh cilantro or parsley leaves for garnish

1. Heat the oven to 400°F.
2. Warm the beans in a large pot with the liquid; add salt and pepper. Adjust the heat so the mixture bubbles very slowly.
3. Bring the oil in a large, deep skillet to medium-high heat. Brown the chicken well on all sides, about 15 minutes; season with salt and pepper, transfer to a roasting pan, and put in the oven.
4. Pour off all but 3 tablespoons of the fat remaining in the skillet. Turn the heat down to medium and add the onion, celery, and carrot. Cook, stirring occasionally, until the vegetables are softened, about 10 minutes.
5. Add the garlic, ginger, coriander, cumin, and tomato and cook for 5 minutes more, stirring occasionally and scraping the bottom of the pan to loosen any brown bits. Add the mixture to the simmering beans.
6. When the chicken has cooked for about 15 minutes, check for doneness. (If the chicken is cooked throughout, the juices will run clear if you make a small cut in the meat near the bone.) When it is ready, remove it from the oven.
7. When the vegetables are tender, put the chickpeas and the vegetables on a large, deep platter. Top with the chicken, garnish, and serve.

¶ MARK BITTMAN'S CHILI NON CARNE

Yield: 6 to 8 servings

This recipe is adapted from noted American food journalist Mark Bittman's How to Cook Everything. *He says that he thinks of chili as "slow-cooked red beans seasoned with cumin and chilis," not as the various dishes made with meat. You can vary this dish with other beans or combinations of beans. Mark recommends trying red, pink, white, pinto, and cannellini beans. Serve with rice, corn tortillas, or whole-grain crackers, and bottled hot sauce for a full meal.*

1 pound dried pinto beans, washed, picked over, and soaked if you like

1 whole yellow or white onion, unpeeled, plus 1 small yellow or white onion, minced
Salt and freshly ground black pepper
1 cup vegetable broth or water
1 fresh hot chili, such as a serrano or a small jalapeño, seeded and minced, or
    to taste (optional)
1 teaspoon ground cumin (optional or to taste)
1 teaspoon minced fresh oregano leaves or ½ teaspoon dried oregano (optional)
1 tablespoon minced garlic
Chopped fresh cilantro for garnish

1. Put the soaked beans in a large pot with water to cover and bring to a boil over high heat, skimming the foam if necessary. Add the whole onion.
2. Adjust the heat so the beans bubble steadily but not violently and cover loosely. Check to be sure you do not boil away all the liquid.
3. When the beans begin to soften (30 minutes to an hour, depending on the type of bean), season with salt and pepper.
4. Continue to cook, stirring occasionally and adding water if necessary, until the beans are quite tender but still intact (about as long as it took them to begin to soften).
5. Drain the beans, reserving the cooking liquid if you choose to use it. Discard the onion and add all the remaining ingredients except the cilantro. Turn the heat to medium and bring to a boil. Cover and turn the heat down to low.
6. Cook, stirring occasionally and adding more liquid if necessary, until the beans are very tender and the flavors have mellowed, about 15 minutes. Taste, adjusting the seasoning, if necessary.
7. Dish up into serving bowls and garnish with cilantro.

Tip: For a slightly different chili taste, try this spice mixture in your beans: 2 teaspoons sweet paprika, 1 teaspoon ground ancho chili pepper, 1 teaspoon cumin, 1 teaspoon ground coriander, 1 teaspoon dried Mexican oregano.

RECIPES FROM IKARIA

¶¶ IKARIAN TEAS

Yield: 1 serving

I believe herbal teas explain Ikaria's low rates of dementia. Depending on the time of year, people here will hike out into the fields and pick fresh herbs. But you can make your own version with dried herbs at home.

1 teaspoon fresh or dried marjoram, sage, and mint leaves
1 tablespoon honey, preferably Ikarian (a dark brown tree and herb honey—optional)
1 lemon wedge (optional)
Up to 2 teaspoons soy creamer (optional)

1. Bring 2 cups water to a simmer in a tea kettle or a small pot set over high heat until bubbles float to the surface or you see strings of small bubbles from the bottom of the kettle. Do not boil. Pour into a cup.
2. Put the herbs in a tea infuser or into an individual tea bag, set in the mug, and steep until well perfumed, 5 to 10 minutes. If desired, sweeten with honey, garnish with a lemon wedge, and/or stir in a splash of soy creamer.

ΥΙ THEA'S GREEK SALAD

Yield: 4 servings

This meal-in-one vegetarian salad is about as good as it gets. Serve it with sourdough bread to dip in olive oil.

2 tablespoons red wine vinegar
1 teaspoon Dijon mustard
¼ cup extra-virgin olive oil
½ teaspoon dried ground rosemary
½ teaspoon salt
½ teaspoon freshly ground black pepper
8 cups field greens, such as a packaged mesclun mix or a mix of baby greens like arugula, kale, baby, or red leaf lettuce
3 medium red globe, beefsteak, or heirloom tomatoes, cut into wedges
1 (12¾-ounce) can artichoke hearts packed in water, drained and cut into quarters
8 cooked and drained small creamer or white potatoes, cut in half (optional)
1 cup soaked, cooked, and drained chickpeas or drained and rinsed canned chickpeas
1 large red bell pepper, stemmed, cored, and cut into ¼-inch-thick strips
1 small cucumber, sliced into ¼-inch-thick rounds
1 small red onion, sliced into paper-thin rings
¼ cup fresh mint leaves
1 teaspoon dried oregano
Kalamata olives, for garnish
Crumbled feta cheese, for garnish
4 hard-cooked eggs, peeled and quartered (optional)

1. Whisk the vinegar and mustard in a large salad bowl until creamy. Whisk in the oil in a slow, steady stream; whisk in the rosemary, salt, and pepper until uniform.
2. Add the field greens, tomatoes, artichoke hearts, potatoes (if using), chickpeas, bell pepper, cucumber, onion, mint leaves, and oregano. Toss gently but well to coat.
3. Divide the salad onto 4 serving plates. Garnish each helping with 3 or 4 olives and about 1 tablespoon crumbled feta. If desired, lay hard-cooked egg quarters around the salads.

Tip: Chill the serving plates in the fridge for 8 hours for an appealing, summery flare.

Tip: To make hard-cooked eggs, set the eggs in a large saucepan and fill three-quarters full with cool tap water. Bring to a simmer over high heat and boil for 1 minute. Cover and set aside off the heat for 5 minutes. Drain, rinse with cool water, and peel quickly while warm.

⅞ HORTA – LONGEVITY GREENS

Yield: 3 to 4 servings

Hortogagos is Greek for vegetarian. Loosely translated, it means "weed eater." On Ikaria, cooked greens are synonymous with weeds—that is, wild greens. And with more than 150 different varieties of edible greens growing on the island, it's no wonder Ikarians eat them most days. They often reserve the cooking water to make tea with lemon. (You can also freeze the cooking water to use as a vegetable broth.) You don't have to forage in the nearest field to enjoy horta. *Your local supermarket or farmers market offers many choices. These qualify as among the world's healthiest foods.*

8 cups mixed leafy greens, such as spinach, dandelion greens, chard, mustard greens, turnip greens, collards, kale, escarole, or beet greens, small leaves left whole or large leaves roughly chopped
⅓ cup extra-virgin olive oil
3 tablespoons fresh lemon juice
¼ teaspoon salt
¼ teaspoon freshly ground black pepper

1. Submerge and agitate the greens in a large bowl of cold water. Set aside for a few minutes, then lift the greens out with tongs or your cleaned hands, leaving the water and any sediment behind. Repeat until there's no sand or grit in the bowl.
2. Bring a large pot of water to a boil over high heat. Add the greens, submerge with a wooden spoon, and cook, uncovered, until wilted, just a minute or two.

3. Drain in a large colander set in the sink, reserving some of the water to make tea, if desired. Transfer to a serving platter or bowl. Drizzle with olive oil and lemon, then season with salt and pepper to serve.

Tip: Collard greens, as well as large leaves of mustard greens, turnip greens, and kale, should be stemmed before cooking.

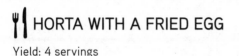 HORTA WITH A FRIED EGG

<u>Yield: 4 servings</u>

Cooked greens, as above
1 tablespoon olive oil
4 large eggs

1. Make horta according to the above recipe.
2. Warm the oil in a large nonstick skillet set over medium heat. Crack an egg into a small bowl or ramekin; slip the egg into the skillet. Repeat with the remaining eggs. Cook until the whites are set and a bit brown around the edges, 2 to 3 minutes. If desired, flip with a nonstick-safe spatula and cook for 1 to 2 minutes, based on your preference for a soft or hard yolk.
3. Divide the cooked greens among four plates and top each with 1 cooked egg.

Tip: For poached eggs, bring a medium saucepan of water to a boil over high heat. Turn off the heat, then crack the eggs into the saucepan, using the ramekin method above. Set aside off the heat for 5 minutes. Use a slotted spoon to drain and transfer the eggs to the horta.

GREEK POTATO SALAD

<u>Yield: 6 servings</u>

This chunky salad of red potatoes, fresh greens, and a couple of boldly flavored herbs reminds me of summer in Ikaria. It's an ideal lunch!

1½ pounds medium red potatoes, peeled and quartered
½ teaspoon celery seeds
½ cup extra-virgin olive oil
2 tablespoons red wine vinegar
1 tablespoon packed fresh oregano leaves, minced
½ teaspoon salt

¼ teaspoon freshly ground black pepper
1 small red leaf lettuce head, cored and chopped (about 3 cups)
2 cups arugula, chopped
½ cup packed fresh mint leaves
Finely chopped scallions, for garnish
Toasted sliced almonds, for garnish
3 hard-cooked eggs (see tip, page 246), peeled and sliced lengthwise (optional)

1. Place the potatoes in a large saucepan. Add enough cool water so they're submerged by 2 inches. Bring to a boil over high heat, then reduce the heat to medium and simmer until firm but easily pierced with a fork, about 15 minutes. Drain in a colander set in the sink and transfer to a large salad bowl; sprinkle the celery seeds over the potatoes while they're hot. Cool for at least 15 minutes or up to 1 hour.

2. Whisk the oil, vinegar, oregano, salt, and pepper in a small bowl until uniform. Pour about a third of this dressing over the potatoes and toss well. The recipe can be completed through this step up to 3 hours in advance. Cover and refrigerate the potatoes until you're ready to make the salad; cover and set the dressing aside at room temperature.

3. Add the lettuce, arugula, and mint leaves to the potatoes. Top with the remainder of the dressing. Toss gently but well. Divide onto 6 serving plates. Garnish each with chopped scallions and about 1 tablespoon toasted sliced almonds for garnish. If desired, place hard-boiled egg slices on the side of each plate.

¶ IKARIAN STEW

Yield: 4 servings

This is hands-down my favorite longevity recipe. This savory one-pot meal fuses the iconic flavors of Ikaria with the faintest hint of sweet fennel. As is customary in Ikaria, a small amount of olive oil is used to sauté the vegetables, then a generous drizzle finishes the dish. This practice is instinctively brilliant: Heat breaks down the oil, so saving most for a final drizzle assures its rich flavor and maximum health benefits. This protein-rich stew freezes well, though the kale will lose a little of its vibrancy. To refresh, add a few more slivered leaves when reheating.

2 cups dried black-eyed peas
½ cup extra-virgin olive oil
1 large yellow or white onion, diced (about 1½ cups)
1 medium fennel bulb, trimmed, halved, and sliced into thin strips
2 teaspoons minced garlic
3 large carrots, peeled and chopped (about 1 cup)

1 large red globe, beefsteak, or heirloom tomato, diced (about ¾ cup)
2 tablespoons tomato paste
2 bay leaves
1 teaspoon salt
4 large kale leaves, slivered
½ cup chopped fresh dill

1. Spread the black-eyed peas on a large baking sheet and pick over to remove any damaged peas or debris. Put the peas in a large pot, add enough cool tap water to submerge by 2 inches, and bring to a boil over high heat. Boil for 1 minute. Set aside off the heat and soak for 1 hour. Drain in a colander set in the sink.
2. Warm ¼ cup oil in a large pot or Dutch oven set over medium heat. Add the onion and fennel; cook, stirring often, until soft, about 8 minutes. Add the garlic and cook until fragrant, about 20 seconds. Stir in the black-eyed peas, carrots, tomato, tomato paste, bay leaves, and salt until the tomato paste dissolves. Add enough water just to cover the vegetables. Raise the heat to medium-high and bring to a boil.
3. Cover, reduce the heat to low, and simmer slowly until the black-eyed peas are tender (not rocklike but not mush), about 50 minutes.
4. Stir in the kale leaves and dill. Cover and cook until the kale is tender, 5 to 10 minutes. Discard the bay leaves. Ladle into four bowls. Drizzle 1 tablespoon olive oil on top of each helping.

Tip: For a quicker meal, substitute 4 cups frozen black-eyed peas, thawed, or 4 cups drained and rinsed canned black-eyed peas—and skip step 1. Simmer the stew in step 3 for only 25 minutes to blend the flavors and cook the fennel. Complete step 4 as directed.

Tip: When working with high-acid foods like tomatoes or vinegar, always cook in nonreactive cookware, such as stainless-steel, anodized aluminum, or enameled cast-iron pans, pots, and skillets.

¶¶ SOUFIKO (IKARIAN RATATOUILLE)

Yield: 4 servings as a main course or 6 to 8 as a side dish

Ikarians' fondness for olive oil is best illustrated in this staple that is made in practically every household on the island, especially during the summer when these vegetables abound. Soufiko is reminiscent of a French ratatouille, except it includes potatoes and some of Ikaria's favorite herbs. It's eaten as a side dish or as a vegetarian meal. The secret to melding the flavors is keeping it at a long, slow simmer as the vegetables cook in the olive oil and their juices. The flavors even intensify over the next day or so, so you can cook it, keep it refrigerated for a day or two, and reheat it at will. By the way, soufiko can be served hot or cold.

10 tablespoons extra-virgin olive oil, plus more for a garnish
2 medium eggplants (about 12 ounces each), stemmed and cut into 1-inch chunks (do not peel)
2 large red potatoes (about 6 ounces each), scrubbed and cut into 1-inch chunks (do not peel)
2 medium yellow or white onions, halved and sliced into thin half-moons
2 tablespoons minced garlic
2 medium red bell peppers (or 1 red and 1 green bell pepper), stemmed, cored, and cut into 1-inch squares
2 medium zucchini (about 5 ounces each), cut into ¼-inch-thick rounds
3 large red globe, beefsteak, or heirloom tomatoes, coarsely chopped (about 2¼ cups)
¼ cup packed fresh oregano leaves, roughly chopped
2 tablespoons packed fresh sage leaves, roughly chopped
1 teaspoon salt
3 tablespoons fresh lemon juice

1. Pour 2 tablespoons olive oil in the bottom of a large pot or Dutch oven. Layer the eggplant, potatoes, onions, garlic, bell peppers, zucchini, and tomatoes in the order listed. Sprinkle the top with half the oregano, all the sage, and the salt. Pour the remaining olive oil (½ cup) evenly over everything.
2. Set the pot over medium heat until the vegetables begin to sizzle in the oil. Cover, reduce the heat to low, and cook for 15 minutes. Stir well and continue cooking, covered, until the vegetables are tender, about 15 more minutes.
3. Sprinkle with the remaining oregano and the lemon juice. Drizzle with a little extra-virgin olive oil as a garnish to serve.

Tip: For a slightly more refined dish, seed the tomatoes. Cut them into quarters, then gently squeeze over the sink, picking out any seeds that remain behind. Now chop these quarters.

Tip: For an extravagant garnish, sprinkle flaked sea salt over each serving.

¶¶ MAGEIRIO – CHUNKY VEGETABLE STEW

<u>Yield: 6 servings</u>

Try this Ikarian combination of vegetables as a summer lunch or an easy dinner any time of year. You won't miss the meat.

2 tablespoons extra-virgin olive oil, plus more for garnish

2 medium yellow or white onions, chopped (about 2 cups)

1 pound fresh green beans, trimmed

3 medium red potatoes (about 4 ounces each), quartered (do not peel)

3 medium zucchini (about 5 ounces each), halved crosswise, then halved lengthwise

3 medium red globe, beefsteak, or heirloom tomatoes, coarsely chopped (about 2 cups)

3 corn ears, husked, the silks removed, and the ears broken in half

1 medium eggplant (about 12 ounces), stemmed and cut into six equal pieces

½ teaspoon salt

3 Italian sweet long peppers, such as cubanel or Italian frying peppers, stemmed, cored, and quartered lengthwise

1. Warm the oil in a large pot or Dutch oven set over medium heat. Add the onions and cook, stirring often, until soft but not brown, about 8 minutes.
2. Stir in the green beans, potatoes, zucchini, tomatoes, corn, eggplant, and salt. Put the long peppers on top. Pour 1 cup water over the vegetables.
3. Bring to a simmer, then reduce the heat to low, cover, and cook, shaking the pan frequently without stirring, until the vegetables are tender, about 45 minutes. Drizzle with olive oil as a garnish to serve.

¶¶ BAKED IKARIAN CHICKPEAS

Yield: 6 servings as a side dish

Ikarians eat a variation of the Mediterranean diet, with lots of fruits and vegetables, whole grains, beans, potatoes, and olive oil—which contains cholesterol-lowering mono-unsaturated fats. Try these delicious baked chickpeas. And don't forget the olive oil!

1 pound dried chickpeas

1 medium zucchini (about 5 ounces), diced

2 medium carrots, peeled and diced (about ½ cup)

1 small yellow or white onion, diced (about ½ cup)

½ cup extra-virgin olive oil

2 tablespoons packed fresh mint leaves, minced

½ teaspoon salt

¼ teaspoon freshly ground black pepper

1. Soak the chickpeas in a big bowl of water at room temperature for at least 8 hours or up to 16 hours (that is, overnight).
2. Drain in a colander set in the sink. Pour the chickpeas into a large saucepan and add enough cool water so they're submerged by 2 inches. Bring to a boil over high heat. Boil for 5 minutes, then drain in a colander set in the sink.
3. Return the chickpeas to the pot, cover with the same amount of fresh water, and bring back to a boil over high heat. Cover, reduce the heat to low, and cook until tender, about 45 minutes. Scoop out 1 cup cooking liquid and set aside. Drain the remainder in a colander set in the sink.
4. Position the rack in the center of the oven and heat the oven to 350°F.
5. Stir the zucchini, carrots, onion, olive oil, and mint in a large roasting pan. Pour the drained chickpeas evenly over the vegetables; pour in the reserved 1 cup cooking liquid.
6. Roast undisturbed until the vegetables are tender and the chickpeas are lightly browned, about 15 minutes. Stir in the salt and pepper. Set aside at room temperature for 5 minutes to blend the flavors before serving.

¶¶ CABBAGE WITH RICE

Yield: 4 servings

The tavern at Thea's Inn is the social hub of eastern Ikaria and my favorite spot to relax while I am there. Athina Mazari, chef at the tavern, cooks this up for me whenever I'm in the area. It's a meal in itself.

2 tablespoons extra-virgin olive oil
1 small green cabbage (about 12 ounces), cored and cut into 1½-inch chunks
2 medium yellow or white onions, coarsely chopped (about 2 cups)
3 large carrots, peeled and grated through the large holes of a box grater
1 cup chopped fresh dill fronds
2 cups vegetable broth
1 cup uncooked long-grain white rice, such as white basmati rice
½ teaspoon salt
¼ teaspoon freshly ground black pepper
Lemon wedges, for garnish

1. Warm the oil in a large saucepan or Dutch oven set over medium heat. Add the cabbage, onions, carrots, and dill; cook, stirring often, until the vegetables begin to soften, about 20 minutes.
2. Add the broth and rice; bring to a simmer. Cover, reduce the heat to low, and simmer slowly until the rice and vegetables are tender, about 20 minutes.

If rice is not done and dish is dry, add a bit of water and continue cooking, covered, for 5 minutes.
3. Stir in the salt and pepper. Divide among 4 plates and serve with lemon wedges for squeezing the juice on top to brighten the flavors.

Tip: You can make this dish with medium-grain white rice (such as arborio). Or you can substitute long-grain brown rice, such as brown basmati; in this case, increase the broth to 2½ cups and increase the cooking time to 45 minutes.

▼▐ IKARIAN BAKED FISH

<u>Yield: 6 servings</u>

John Dory, bronzino, dorado, bream, and goatfish are just a few of the fish you might find in Ikarian fish markets. Any of these fish can be used in this dish, as well as tilefish (a great source of omega-3s), flounder, or red snapper. It is customarily served with horta.

2 large red potatoes (about 6 ounces each), sliced into ¼-inch-thick rounds (do not peel)
6 (5- to 6-ounce) white-fleshed fish fillets, such as any in the headnote, skinned
½ teaspoon salt
½ teaspoon freshly ground black pepper
2 large yellow or white onions, sliced into ¼-inch-thick rings
2 large red globe, beefsteak, or heirloom tomatoes, cut into ¼-inch-thick rounds
3 garlic cloves, peeled and thinly sliced
2 large carrots, peeled, halved crosswise, then sliced into ¼-inch-thick strips lengthwise
1 cup dry white wine, such as Afianes begleri, Ktima Pavlidis Thema, or an unoaked California chardonnay
½ cup extra-virgin olive oil
½ cup packed fresh parsley leaves, chopped
1 tablespoon dried oregano
6 tablespoons fresh lemon juice

1. Position the rack in the center of the oven and heat the oven to 375°F.
2. Set the potato rings in an even layer in the bottom of a 9 x 13-inch baking dish. Top with the fillets; season with salt and pepper. Cover evenly with the onion rings, then layer the tomato rings over the onions. Sprinkle the garlic on top. Place the carrots around the sides of the dish. Pour the wine and olive oil over the casserole; sprinkle with the parsley and oregano.

3. Bake uncovered until the fish is cooked through and the vegetables are tender, about 30 minutes.
4. Pour the lemon juice over the casserole and set aside for 5 minutes on a wire rack at room temperature to blend the flavors before serving. Dish into bowls or onto plates with a large spoon or spatula to keep the fillets intact.

¶¶ IKARIAN-STYLE SOURDOUGH BREAD

Yield: Starter and 1 loaf

On my many visits to Ikaria, I tasted the most wonderful bread made with starter dough containing local bacteria rather than conventional yeast. But you don't need Ikarian bacteria to make sourdough bread. Start by making the starter dough, which is more of an art than a science. Temperature, humidity, altitude, and locale can all affect it, so you may need to make some adjustments to the recipe shared below. Experience counts too, so if at first you don't succeed, try again until you get the hang of it.

For the starter:
1 (0.24-ounce) package dry live-culture yeast-free sourdough starter for wheat flour, such as Desem
2 cups bread flour, or more as necessary
For the loaf:
4 to 6 cups bread flour
Canola or vegetable oil, for greasing the baking sheet

1. Make the starter based on the instructions given in or on the packet. In general, you'll mix a small amount of nonchlorinated water (such as bottled spring water) with the starter, then feed it small amounts of flour over the course of several days until bubbling with a distinctly fermented aroma.
2. Place 2 cups prepared starter in a large bowl; stir in 2 cups lukewarm nonchlorinated water. Stir in 4 cups bread flour until a soft dough forms, adding more flour in ¼-cup increments until the dough can be gathered into a coherent, not sticky ball. (Place the excess starter in a separate bowl and continue to feed with nonchlorinated water and small amounts of flour every few days as directed by the package to preserve for another baking.)
3. Lightly flour a clean, dry work surface. Set the ball of dough on it and knead until elastic and very smooth, about 20 minutes, adding more flour in 1-tablespoon increments only if the dough seems sticky. Gather back into a ball, place in a large bowl, cover with a clean kitchen towel, and set aside in a warm, draft-free place until doubled in bulk, between 6 and 12 hours. (Do not stint on the time.)

4. Plunge your cleaned fist into the dough to deflate it. Turn out onto a dry, cleaned, lightly floured work surface and knead lightly for 1 minute. Shape into a free form, round or oval loaf about 10 inches in diameter or at the oval's longest point.

5. Lightly grease a large, lipped baking sheet and transfer the loaf to it. Cover with a clean kitchen towel and set aside in a warm, draft-free place until doubled in bulk, 4 to 8 hours. Meanwhile, position the rack in the center of the oven and heat the oven to 350°F.

6. Bake until browned and hollow sounding when tapped, about 1 hour. Transfer to a wire baking rack and cool for at least 10 minutes or up to 2 hours before slicing to serve.

Tip: For an easier preparation, knead the dough in the bowl of a stand mixer with the dough hook at low speed in step 3.

Tip: A second rising yields an exceptionally sour bread. However, you can skip this step. If so, knead the bread as directed in step 3, skip the first rising and all of step 4, then form the dough into the desired shape, letting it rise one time only as directed in step 5.

RECIPES FROM OKINAWA

¶¶ MISO SOUP WITH VEGETABLES

Yield: 4 servings

Though miso soup is usually considered an appetizer for lunch or dinner in American Japanese restaurants, Okinawan centenarian Kamada Nakazato preferred to eat it for breakfast, spiked with vegetables she picked from her garden. In the United States, miso and fresh shiitake mushrooms are available in Asian markets and many mainstream supermarkets. Darker miso has a stronger flavor and is saltier than lighter white to yellow miso (considered the general purpose miso).

3 tablespoons miso paste, such as *shiro miso* (white), *miso* (aka red miso), or *shinshu miso* (yellow)

1½ tablespoons unseasoned rice wine vinegar

1 large garlic clove, peeled

1½-inch fresh ginger piece, peeled

½ pound firm tofu, cut into ½-inch cubes

¼ pound fresh shiitake mushrooms, stemmed and the caps thinly sliced

2 cups pea shoots (about 3 ounces), roughly chopped
6 medium scallions, trimmed and thinly chopped
2 teaspoons toasted sesame oil
1 teaspoon soy sauce

1. Put the miso, rice vinegar, garlic, ginger, and 1 cup water in a food processor or a large blender. Cover and process or blend until smooth, scraping down the inside of the canister at least once.
2. Stir the miso mixture into 4 additional cups water in a medium saucepan. Add the tofu, mushrooms, pea shoots, and scallions; bring to a simmer over medium heat, stirring often. Reduce the heat to low and simmer, uncovered, for 5 minutes. Turn off heat and stir in the sesame oil and soy sauce before serving.

Tip: If you like more texture, finely mince the garlic and ginger but don't put them in the food processor or blender. Instead, add them with the tofu in step 2.

Tip: If fresh shiitake mushrooms are not available, soak 4 large dried shiitakes with warm tap water in a small bowl for 20 minutes. Drain, reserving the soaking liquid. Strain the liquid through cheesecloth to remove grit. Use this soaking liquid, reducing the amount of water in the saucepan by an equivalent amount.

Tip: Substitute baby spinach or stemmed watercress for the pea shoots.

￮￮ COCONUT-MASHED SWEET POTATOES

Yield: 6 servings as a side dish

Imo *means sweet potato in Japanese, and in Okinawa it refers to the purple sweet potato, which was the basic staple of the Okinawan diet in the early years of the 20th century and after World War II. The orange-fleshed sweet potatoes we are accustomed to make a fine substitute.*

5 medium sweet potatoes (about 3 pounds), peeled and cut into 1-inch cubes
Up to ¾ cup regular or low-fat canned coconut milk
1 teaspoon ground cinnamon, or more as necessary
½ teaspoon salt, optional

1. Place the sweet potatoes in a large pot and add enough water so they're submerged by 1 inch. Bring to a boil over high heat, then reduce the heat to medium and cook until the potatoes are soft, about 25 minutes.
2. Drain in a colander set in the sink, then transfer the sweet potatoes to a large bowl. Add ½ cup coconut milk and mash with a potato masher or

an electric mixer at medium-low speed until creamy, adding more coconut milk to get a smooth, rich puree. Stir in the cinnamon, as well as the salt, if desired.

Tip: For a different taste and lower fat, substitute half the coconut milk for fresh orange juice while mashing. Remember to add the ground cinnamon!

¶¶ "STONE"-BAKED SWEET POTATOES

Yield: 4 servings

Baking Okinawan purple sweet potatoes or our orange-fleshed ones results in a rich taste and smooth texture that melts in your mouth. Many Okinawans still enjoy "stone"-baked potatoes from vendors who sell them from little trucks. You can enjoy similar goodness by baking sweet potatoes in your oven. Using a pizza stone or cast-iron skillet will add the stone-baked touch.

4 medium sweet potatoes (about 10 ounces each)
Aluminum foil
Salt, for garnish
Ground cinnamon, for garnish

1. Position the rack in the center of the oven and heat the oven to 350°F.
2. Line a cast-iron skillet or broiler pan with foil—or lay a sheet of foil on a pizza stone or a baking sheet and turn the foil up 1 inch on all sides to form a lip that can stop oozing juices.
3. Bake for 25 minutes, then turn the sweet potatoes over, protecting your hand with a pot holder or folded dry kitchen towel. Continue baking until the sweet potatoes are soft to the touch, about 20 more minutes. The longer the cooking time, the more the juice caramelizes next to the potato skin, which is the way many Okinawans like their baked potatoes. Cool for a few minutes, then slit the skin lengthwise. Although not necessary, you can garnish with a pinch of salt or ground cinnamon.

¶¶ SOMEN NOODLES WITH STEAMED VEGETABLES

Yield: 4 servings

Somen *noodles are thin delicate Japanese noodles that cook up quickly. (Don't confuse them with soba noodles.) Somen noodles are often served cold.*

¼ cup soy sauce, preferably a Japanese bottling
¼ cup mirin
2 teaspoons toasted sesame oil
1 teaspoon Asian red chili paste, such as *sambal oelek*
1 teaspoon minced garlic
½ teaspoon minced peeled fresh ginger
14 ounces dried somen noodles
1 cup julienned green pepper
1 cup julienned carrot
1 cup shredded green cabbage
Thinly sliced scallions, for garnish

1. Whisk the soy sauce, mirin, sesame oil, chili paste, garlic, and ginger in a large bowl.
2. Cook the somen noodles in a large saucepan of water according to the package directions. Drain in a colander set in the sink and rinse with cool water to stop the cooking. Drain well, add to the soy sauce mixture, and toss gently.
3. Bring about ¼ cup water to a boil in the same saucepan that had cooked the noodles. Add the green peppers, carrots, and cabbage; cover, reduce the heat to low, and cook until soft, about 3 minutes. Drain in that colander; rinse with cool tap water to chill. Drain well, shaking the colander over the sink a few times.
4. Add the vegetables to the noodles and sauce; toss well. Serve at once or cover and refrigerate for up to 4 hours. Garnish with sliced scallions before serving.

Tip: Mirin is a sweet, Japanese rice wine that is often used in cooking. It is available in the international aisle of almost all North American supermarkets. But if you can't find it, substitute ¼ cup dry white wine and 2 teaspoons sugar. If you prefer no alcohol in the dish, substitute unsweetened grape juice (without adding any sugar).

ᵠᶦ MUSHROOM STEW

Yield: 4 servings

Asian markets that cater to a Japanese clientele have an enormous variety of mushrooms, but many types of Japanese mushrooms are available at most local supermarkets. Just make sure to include shiitakes in the mix.

2½ pounds assorted Japanese mushrooms, such as stemmed shiitake caps, maitake, and trimmed enoki

1 cup dry sake or dry white wine, such as pinot gris
1 cup vegetable broth
2 tablespoons soy sauce, preferably a Japanese bottling
1 tablespoon oyster sauce
1 teaspoon tomato paste
1 teaspoon Asian red chili paste, such as *sambal oelek*
3 tablespoons peanut oil, sesame oil, or extra-virgin olive oil
4 medium shallots, peeled and diced
2 tablespoons minced garlic
1 teaspoon dried thyme, optional
1 bay leaf
2 cups cooked long- or medium-grain brown rice

1. Wipe the mushrooms clean with a damp paper towel and cut them into 1-inch pieces and set aside. Whisk the wine, broth, soy sauce, oyster sauce, tomato paste, and chili paste in a small bowl and set aside.
2. Warm the oil in a large sauté pan or a deep skillet set over medium heat. Add the shallots and garlic; cook, stirring often, until lightly browned, about 2 minutes. Add the mushrooms and stir until all the oil has been absorbed. Pour in the wine mixture; stir in the thyme and bay leaf.
3. Raise the heat to medium-high and bring to a simmer. Reduce the heat to low and continue cooking, uncovered, until the liquid in the pan has reduced to half its original volume, 15 to 20 minutes.
4. Pile the rice on a large serving platter. Spoon the mushroom stew on top, using the pan juices as a sauce.

Tip: If you want to omit the sake or wine, increase the broth to 2 cups.

Tip: A little dried thyme isn't traditional, but it will offer a slightly herbaceous flavor among the sweeter notes in the stew.

Tip: You can also serve this stew with "yellow rice" by adding up to 1 teaspoon ground dried turmeric to the rice's cooking water.

¶¶ TOFU AND BOK CHOY STIR-FRY

Yield: 4 servings

This dish is traditionally made with mizuna, a peppery Japanese leafy green, but arugula makes a nice substitute if you can't find it. I also substitute olive oil for the traditional peanut oil. If you want, serve this easy stir-fry over cooked brown rice.

1 (12-ounce) block extra-firm tofu
¼ cup soy sauce, preferably a Japanese bottling
1 tablespoon toasted sesame oil
1 tablespoon unseasoned rice vinegar
3 tablespoons peanut oil or extra-virgin olive oil
6 medium scallions, trimmed and thinly sliced
1½ tablespoons minced garlic
1 tablespoon minced peeled fresh ginger
4 small bok choy (about 8 ounces total weight), the leaves separated and rinsed
   to remove grit
4 cups loosely packed mizuna or baby arugula

1. Wrap the tofu block in paper towels and gently squeeze out excess moisture. You may also place the wrapped tofu block on a shallow plate and then top the tofu with a second plate and a weight, such as a can of vegetables, and set aside for 5 to 10 minutes to remove the moisture.
2. Unwrap the tofu and cut crosswise into ½-inch slices, then cut each slice in half crosswise; set aside. Whisk the soy sauce, sesame oil, and vinegar in a small bowl; set aside.
3. Set a large nonstick wok or nonstick skillet over medium-high heat for a couple minutes, then swirl in 2 tablespoons of the oil. Add the tofu and cook until golden brown, turning once, about 4 minutes. Transfer to a paper towel–lined plate to drain.
4. Pour the remaining tablespoon of oil into the wok or skillet. Add the scallions, garlic, and ginger; stir-fry until fragrant, about 30 seconds. Add the bok choy leaves and half of the soy sauce mixture. Stir-fry until the bok choy wilts, about 2 minutes. Add the mizuna or arugula and toss until it wilts, less than 1 minute. Return the tofu to the wok and add the remaining soy sauce mixture. Toss until heated through, less than 1 minute.

Tip: For peanut allergies, substitute soybean or canola oil.

¶¶ GRILLED TOFU WITH SHIITAKE MUSHROOMS

Yield: 4 servings

Though Okinawans love their pork, it is traditionally served only on special occasions. Mostly, their diet is vegetarian with a lot of tofu. This is what an everyday meal might look like.

2 (12-ounce) blocks extra-firm tofu

¼ cup all-purpose flour
½ teaspoon salt
¼ teaspoon freshly ground black pepper
2 tablespoons peanut oil or extra-virgin olive oil
2 medium shallots, peeled and minced
½ pound shiitake mushroom caps, thinly sliced
1 tablespoon soy sauce
1 tablespoon dry sake or moderately dry white wine, such as pinot gris

1. Gently squeeze the excess moisture from the tofu blocks, following the instructions in step 1 of the previous recipe. Cut the tofu crosswise into 1-inch-thick slices.
2. Whisk the flour, salt, and pepper on a large plate. Dredge the tofu pieces in the seasoned flour and shake lightly to remove any excess. Set aside on a cutting board.
3. Warm 1 tablespoon of the oil in a large nonstick skillet set over medium heat. Add the tofu slices and cook until golden brown, turning once, about 4 minutes. Transfer to a serving platter.
4. Add the remaining 1 tablespoon of oil to the skillet. Add the shallots and cook, stirring often, until softened, about 1 minute. Add the mushrooms and stir until wilted, about 2 minutes. Mix in the soy sauce and sake or wine. Stir until the vegetables are coated in the sauce, then spoon over the tofu to serve.

¶❘ GOYA CHAMPURU (BITTER MELON STIR-FRY)

Yield: 4 servings

The island's iconic dish, goya champuru stars bitter melon, a vegetable that is crunchy and watery like a zucchini but very bitter. You can find bitter melon in Asian markets and in many farmers markets, but you can also substitute cucumbers for a much sweeter flavor. The vegetable is combined with tofu, egg, pork, and onions in a soy-based sauce. Recipes vary from cook to cook. The dish is best made in a cast-iron skillet.

2 small bitter melons (about 8 inches diameter each)
2 teaspoons salt
8 ounces extra-firm tofu
2 tablespoons peanut or canola oil, or more as necessary
3 ounces pork tenderloin, sliced into ¼-inch-thick rounds
1 medium yellow or white onion, halved and sliced into thin half-moons
2 large eggs, well beaten in a small bowl

2 tablespoons soy sauce, preferably a Japanese bottling
2 tablespoons sake, optional

1. Slice the bitter melons lengthwise; use a small spoon to scoop out the hard white core and seeds, leaving a shell of pale green flesh. Slice into ¼-inch-thick half-moons. Toss with the salt in a medium bowl and set aside for 10 minutes. Rinse in a colander set in the sink, then squeeze gently by the handful to remove excess liquid (and thus bitterness). Dry well on paper towels.
2. Wrap the tofu in a paper towel and microwave for 1 minute. Remove from the paper towel and wrap in a clean paper towel for about 10 minutes to absorb more liquid. Cut into ½-inch-thick slices.
3. Heat 1 tablespoon of the oil in a cast-iron pan. Add the pork and brown well, about 3 minutes per side. Transfer to a bowl. Add a little oil if the pan is dry, then add the tofu and brown for about 4 minutes, turning once. Transfer to the bowl with the pork.
4. Pour the remaining 1 tablespoon of oil into the skillet. When hot, add the bitter melon and stir-fry for 1 minute. Add the onion and stir-fry until lightly browned, about 2 minutes. Return the pork and tofu to the pan.
5. Pour in the beaten eggs, cook undisturbed for 10 seconds, then stir gently until scrambled. Pour in the soy sauce and, if using it, the sake. Stir a few seconds to heat through, then serve hot.

Tip: Extra-firm tofu is sometimes sold in small cakes, about 4 ounces each, usually grouped 3 to 5 per package. Two of these cakes would be best for this recipe.

ⅱ LONGEVITY STIR-FRY (GOYA CHAMPLE)

Yield: 4 servings

Chample, *often called* champuru, *means "mixed up" in Okinawan. That seems to me to be an appropriate name for the stir-fry that is the signature dish of Okinawan cooking. The national favorite,* goya champuru *(above), is more of a celebratory dish that includes eggs and pork in addition to bitter melon. This is a more everyday dish: Provided by Craig Willcox, it's an easy-to-fix vegetable chample that is a good way to start exploring Okinawan cuisine. Serve with cooked brown or white rice.*

6 ounces extra-firm tofu
2 tablespoons canola oil
3 cups cored, shredded green cabbage (about 1 small cabbage)
6 ounces green beans (about 1½ cups), trimmed and cut into 2-inch-long pieces

½ cup soybean or mung bean sprouts
2 teaspoons low-sodium soy sauce, preferably a Japanese bottling
¼ teaspoon freshly ground black pepper

1. Gently squeeze excess moisture out of the tofu block (see the microwave technique in step 2 on page 262). Cut the tofu into 1-inch cubes.
2. Warm 1 tablespoon of the oil in a large nonstick skillet set over medium heat. Add the tofu cubes and cook until golden brown, turning occasionally, about 4 minutes. Transfer to a large plate.
3. Add the remaining tablespoon of oil to the skillet. Add the cabbage and green beans; cook, stirring often, until the cabbage begins to wilt, about 3 minutes.
4. Add the bean sprouts and cook, stirring more frequently, for only 1 minute to avoid overcooking. Return the tofu to the skillet and toss gently until heated through, about 1 minute. Stir in the soy sauce, salt, and pepper before serving.

Tip: You can make this simple recipe substituting a variety of vegetables for bean sprouts: zucchini, yellow summer squash, or green or red bell peppers, cored and sliced into 2-inch-long matchsticks. Or substitute Asian cabbage (such as napa or bok choy) for the green cabbage.

Tip: If you like your food a little spicy, add a dash of Okinawan hot sauce, *kore-gusu,* which is made of red peppers and Okinawan sake. Or use the bottled hot sauce of your choice.

¶¶ SHOYU PORK
Yield: 6 servings

Pork belly is simply unsmoked bacon—and long-cooked pork belly is a treasured dish in Okinawa (and one of the best dishes I have ever eaten). The pork is initially simmered in water and skimmed of its fat. Okinawans traditionally simmer it in katsuo dashi, a sweet-savory fish broth, skimming off the fat every few hours until all that remains is an impossibly tender and delicious collagen. Making this dish without the fish broth only slightly alters the flavor. Shoyu is traditionally served with cooked white rice.

1½ pounds pork belly
Parchment paper
½ cup katsuo dashi (recipe follows)
½ cup mirin (see tip, page 258)
½ cup soy sauce, preferably a Japanese bottling
½ cup packed dark brown sugar

1 tablespoon minced peeled fresh ginger
1 tablespoon minced garlic

1. Put the pork in a large pot or Dutch oven and add enough water so it's submerged by 2 inches. Bring to a simmer over high heat. Reduce the heat to medium and cook for 5 minutes. Transfer the pork to a cutting board and discard the water. (Doing this step will cut down on the impurities in the dish as the pork cooks.)
2. Return the pork to the pot; add more fresh water so the meat is again submerged by 2 inches. Bring to a simmer over high heat. Reduce the heat to low, cover, and cook, skimming the surface of the pot frequently for scum and foam, until the pork begins to get tender, about 1 hour.
3. Remove the pork to a cutting board and cool for 10 minutes. Trim the pork of any thick skin and any outer layer of fat. Cut the meat into 1-inch cubes.
4. Wash out the pot or Dutch oven. Cut a piece of parchment paper that will fit inside the pot. Remove the parchment paper and add the katsuo dashi, mirin, soy sauce, brown sugar, ginger, and garlic. Set the pot over high heat and bring to a boil, stirring until the brown sugar dissolves.
5. Add the pork belly pieces and bring to a boil. Reduce the heat to low, lay the parchment paper on the surface of the stew, and simmer until the pork is fork-tender, about 45 minutes, lifting the parchment paper occasionally with kitchen tongs and turning the pork pieces to coat evenly in the sauce. Serve the pork belly with the sauce over cooked white rice.

Tip: If you don't want to make the katsuo dashi, you can substitute water but the flavor of the dish will be less complex.

▓ KATSUO DASHI (JAPANESE FISH STOCK)

Bring ½ cup water to a boil in a small saucepan set over high heat. Stir in ½ cup bonito flakes (found in most Asian markets or online). Reduce the heat to low, cover, and simmer for 5 minutes. Strain through a fine-mesh sieve or a colander lined with cheesecloth or a large coffee filter. Add enough water to make a total volume of ½ cup.

▓ YAKISOBA

Yield: 4 servings

While most Japanese soba noodles are dried buckwheat noodles, Okinawan soba noodles are fresh and made from whole wheat. They're firmer and chewier than the traditional Japanese variety. You might be able to find them in an Asian marketplace or online. However, it is fine to substitute other cooked and drained Japanese soba noodles in this simple recipe. This dish is traditionally made with pork belly, but I substitute pork tenderloin to give it a leaner flavor and a cleaner finish.

½ pound pork tenderloin
3 tablespoons peanut or canola oil
1 medium yellow or white onion, halved and sliced into thin half-moons
4 cups cored and chopped green cabbage (about half a large cabbage)
1 large carrot, peeled and shredded through the large holes of a box grater
2 ounces shiitake mushroom caps, thinly sliced (about 1 cup)
3 tablespoons *yakisoba* sauce or Worcestershire sauce
1 (14-ounce) package Okinawan soba noodles (thawed if frozen)
Pickled sushi ginger, for garnish

1. Slice the pork tenderloin in half crosswise, then cut lengthwise into ½-inch-thick strips. Cut each strip into ½-inch-wide sticks.
2. Warm 2 tablespoons of the oil in a large nonstick wok or skillet set over medium-high heat. Add the pork and onion. Stir-fry until the onions are translucent and the pork has browned on all sides, about 5 minutes. Add the cabbage, carrot, shiitakes, and yakisoba or Worcestershire sauce. Continue to stir-fry until the cabbage begins to wilt, about 2 minutes.
3. Push the pork and vegetables up the sides of the wok so you have a well in the center. Pour the remaining 1 tablespoon of oil in the center of the wok, add the soba noodles, and stir to coat with the oil. Push the pork and vegetables over the noodles, pour ½ cup water on top, cover, and cook undisturbed for 2 minutes. Uncover, toss well, and garnish with pickled sushi ginger.

Tip: Yakisoba sauce is a thick, sweet, and salty condiment, sort of like Japanese barbecue sauce, a favorite on these noodles. Look for it in the international aisle of very large supermarkets, at most Asian markets, and from online suppliers.

Tip: Discard any seasoning packet found with the Okinawan noodles.

RECIPES FROM SARDINIA

¶| MELIS FAMILY MINESTRONE

Yield: 4 servings

This bountiful dish is eaten for lunch every day by the world's longest-lived family, the Melises. Traditionally, it is made with whatever is growing in the garden, but it always includes beans and fregula, *a toasted pebble-size semolina pasta that is popular in Sardinia. Fregula can be purchased at Italian markets or online. If you can't find fregula, any tiny pasta, such as Israeli couscous or acini di pepe, will do. My version also takes a little time to cook. As Gianni Pes points out, a longer cooking time melds the flavors and enhances the bioavailability of more nutrients, such as the lycopene in tomatoes and carotenoids and other antioxidants. A shorter cooking time will make a tasty dish as well, but nutritionally inferior. Traditionally, the minestrone is accompanied with slices of* pane carasau, *or Sardinian flat bread.*

½ cup dried peeled fava beans
½ cup dried cranberry beans
⅓ cup dried chickpeas
7 tablespoons extra-virgin olive oil
1 medium yellow or white onion, chopped (about 1 cup)
2 medium carrots, peeled and chopped (about ⅔ cup)
2 medium celery stalks, chopped (about ½ cup)
2 teaspoons minced garlic
1 (28-ounce) can crushed tomatoes (about 3½ cups)
3 medium yellow potatoes, peeled and diced (about 1½ cups)
1½ cups chopped fennel
¼ cup loosely packed fresh Italian flat-leaf parsley leaves, chopped
2 tablespoons chopped fresh basil leaves
⅔ cup of Sardinian fregula, Israeli couscous, or acini di pepe pasta
½ teaspoon salt
½ teaspoon freshly ground black pepper
¼ cup finely grated pecorino Romano (about 2 ounces)

1. Soak the fava beans, cranberry beans, and chickpeas in a large bowl of water for at least 8 hours or up to 16 hours (that is, overnight). Drain in a colander set in the sink. Rinse well.
2. Warm 3 tablespoons of the olive oil in a large soup pot or Dutch oven set over medium-high heat. Add the onion, carrots, and celery; cook, stirring often, until soft but not browned, about 5 minutes. Add the garlic and cook until fragrant, about 20 seconds.
3. Stir in the tomatoes, potatoes, fennel, parsley, and basil, as well as the drained beans and chickpeas. Add enough water (6 to 8 cups) so that everything is submerged by 1 inch.
4. Raise the heat to high and bring to a full boil. Reduce the heat to low and simmer slowly, uncovered, until the beans are tender, adding more water as necessary if the mixture gets too thick, about 1½ hours.

5. Stir in the pasta, salt, and pepper. Add up to 2 cups water if the soup seems too dry. Continue simmering, uncovered, until the pasta is tender, about 10 minutes.
6. Pour 1 tablespoon of olive oil into each of four serving bowls. Divide the soup among them and top each with 1 tablespoon of the grated cheese.

Tip: You can vary the beans in the minestrone: pinto beans make a good substitute for cranberry beans; great northern or cannellini beans, for the favas.

Tip: Use the stalks and fronds that come off a fennel bulb for the most intense flavor. No feathery fronds on the bulb? Add a teaspoon of fennel seeds to the aromatic vegetables you sauté to begin the dish.

Tip: Add other fresh vegetables from the garden or market, such as zucchini, cabbage, green beans, and cauliflower or broccoli florets.

Tip: Want a stronger tomato taste? Stir in a tablespoon or two of tomato paste. You get the idea!

¶¶ MINESTRA DI FAGIOLI

<u>Yield: 6 servings</u>

This soup, made with beans and whole-grain hulled barley, is often overlooked in favor of the more popular minestrone, made with beans and pasta. The barley enriches the soup with a nutty flavor and more fiber.

1 cup dried great northern beans
½ cup dried hull-less whole-grain barley (not pearled or semi-pearled barley)
6 cups (1½ quarts) vegetable broth
2 medium yellow potatoes, peeled and cut into ½-inch chunks (about 1 cup)
1 medium yellow or white onion, chopped (about 1 cup)
2 medium celery stalks, thinly sliced (about ½ cup)
1 medium carrot, peeled and coarsely chopped (about ¼ cup)
2 teaspoons minced garlic
1 teaspoon dried basil
½ teaspoon ground sage
1 (4-inch) fresh rosemary sprig
1 bay leaf
½ cup loosely packed fresh Italian flat-leaf parsley leaves, chopped
2 tablespoons extra-virgin olive oil
½ teaspoon salt
¼ teaspoon freshly ground black pepper

1. Soak the beans and barley in a large bowl of water at room temperature for 8 hours or up to 12 hours (that is, overnight). Drain in a colander set in the sink and rinse well.
2. Put the beans and barley in a large pot or Dutch oven. Add the broth, potatoes, onion, celery, carrot, garlic, basil, sage, rosemary, and bay leaf. Set over high heat and bring to boil, stirring occasionally.
3. Reduce the heat to low, cover, and simmer slowly until the beans and barley are tender, about 1 hour. Discard the rosemary sprig and bay leaf; stir in the parsley, oil, salt, and pepper before serving.

Tip: To enhance the flavors, sauté the onion, garlic, basil, and sage in 1 tablespoon olive oil until the onion is translucent but not browned, then add to the other ingredients before cooking.

Tip: The soup freezes exceptionally well. Store in sealed, single-serving containers in the freezer for up to 4 months.

¶¶ FAVA BEAN AND MINT SALAD

<u>Yield: 4 servings</u>

Fava beans are synonymous with Sardinia and are often eaten simply out of hand. When fava beans arrive with the debut of spring, large pots go on the stove to cook them quickly and peel them out of their skin. Fava beans and mint are a natural combination.

6 pounds fresh fava beans in the pods or 1 pound fresh fava beans without the pods
1 tablespoon plus ¼ teaspoon salt
2 tablespoons extra-virgin olive oil
1 medium yellow or white onion, diced (about 1 cup)
1 cup loosely packed fresh mint leaves
4 sheets pane *carasau* (Sardinian flat bread) or small pieces of whole-grain flat
   bread (optional)
¼ cup finely grated pecorino Romano (about 2 ounces)

1. To prepare the fava beans, place the 1 tablespoon salt in a large pot, fill it three-quarters full with water, and bring to a boil over high heat. Meanwhile, fill a large bowl with ice water. Drop the beans into the boiling water; cook for 2 minutes. Drain in a colander set in the sink and transfer immediately to the cold water to stop the cooking. Cool for several minutes, then drain in that colander.
2. If you wish to peel the outer layer of the bean, open the skin with your thumbnail at the "eye," where the bean was attached to the pod, and gently squeeze out

the bean. Many Sardinians do not peel fresh fava beans because they enjoy the extra flavor. Test and see which you prefer.

3. Warm the oil in a large skillet set over medium-high heat. Add the onion and cook, stirring often, just until barely softened, about 2 minutes. Add the fava beans and the ¼ teaspoon salt; cook until warmed through, stirring constantly, about 2 minutes.

4. Remove the skillet from the heat. Add the mint and stir well. Put a piece of pane carasau, if you are serving it, on each serving plate. Top each with a quarter of the bean mixture and 1 tablespoon grated cheese.

Tip: Substitute 1 pound frozen fava beans, thawed. Because of the way freezing changes textures, you will probably want to peel each bean after boiling.

¶| TOMATO, ARTICHOKE, AND FENNEL SALAD

<u>Yield: 4 servings</u>

These three vegetables are mainstays of the Sardinian diet and are combined in a variety of dishes—like this one.

2 tablespoons extra-virgin olive oil
2 tablespoons fresh orange juice
1 tablespoon finely grated orange zest
1 tablespoon red wine vinegar
½ teaspoon salt, preferably sea salt
½ teaspoon freshly ground black pepper
2 medium red globe, beefsteak, or heirloom tomatoes (about 8 ounces each), cored and cut into small wedges
2 small fennel bulbs (about 4 ounces each), trimmed and the blemished outer layer removed, then quartered and roughly chopped
1 (14-ounce) can artichoke hearts packed in water, drained and roughly chopped
2 tablespoons packed fresh mint leaves, chopped

1. Whisk the olive oil, orange juice, orange zest, vinegar, salt, and pepper in a large bowl until uniform.

2. Add the tomatoes, fennel, artichokes, and mint leaves. Toss gently to coat.

Tip: To core tomatoes, use a small paring knife to cut out the hard bit where the stem had attached to the fruit.

Tip: If your fennel bulb comes with the fronds and stems, use them in minestrone (page 265) or other soups, stews, or green salads.

¶| SARDINIAN TOMATO SAUCE

<u>Yield: 7 cups</u>

Centenarians make foods from recipes passed down through generations, mixed with their own instinct and, of course, whatever is ripe in the garden. Virtually every Sardinian family has its "secret" tomato sauce. The best ingredient, I am told, is plum tomatoes, which must be skinned and seeded, a time-consuming chore. But this is an authentic Sardinian tomato sauce even with a slight twist: I use canned Italian plum tomatoes that are already skinned and seeded, a real time-saver. It cuts hands-on time to about 10 minutes. Feel free to double or even triple the recipe, because it freezes well in sealed containers for up to 4 months.

¼ cup extra-virgin olive oil
1 large yellow or white onion, diced (about 1 cup)
1 tablespoon minced garlic
2 teaspoons fennel seeds
2 (28-ounce) cans diced seeded plum tomatoes, such as San Marzano tomatoes
    (about 7 cups)
1 large carrot, peeled and broken in half
1 medium celery stalk, broken in half
½ cup chopped fresh basil leaves
2 bay leaves
1 teaspoon salt

1. Warm the oil in a Dutch oven or large pot set over medium heat. Add the onion and cook, stirring often, until soft, about 5 minutes. Do not brown. Add the garlic and fennel seeds; cook until fragrant, about 20 seconds.
2. Add the tomatoes, carrot, celery, basil, bay leaves, and salt. Stir well and bring to a full simmer. Reduce the heat to very low, cover, and simmer slowly for 1 hour. Remove from the heat and cool for 20 minutes.
3. Discard the carrot, celery, and bay leaves. Use an immersion blender to puree the sauce in the pot until smooth and velvety.

Tip: You can also puree the sauce in a large food processor fitted with the chopping blade, although you'll probably have to work in two batches to avoid overflow.

¶| WHITE BEAN SMASH

<u>Yield: About 3 cups</u>

This Italian-style puree is served like a condiment. Its consistency and use are much like chickpea hummus. I put it out on individual small plates with grilled sourdough bread or corn tortillas at dinners instead of bread and butter. Eat it for lunch in corn tortilla wraps with shredded lettuce and chopped fresh tomato or even purchased salsa. It will keep in the refrigerator in a sealed container for up to 5 days.

1½ tablespoons minced garlic
½ teaspoon kosher or coarse salt
3 cups drained and rinsed canned white beans, such as great northern or cannellini
¼ cup extra-virgin olive oil
2 tablespoons fresh lemon juice
Ground rosemary, for garnish
Ground sage, for garnish

1. Place the garlic and salt in a mortar and grind with the pestle until a coarse, grainy paste. Scrape into a large bowl.
2. Add the beans, olive oil, and lemon juice. Use a potato masher to create a thick, smooth, creamy spread.
3. Scrape into a serving bowl or small plates and dust with the rosemary and sage before serving.

Tip: If you don't have a mortar and pestle, process the garlic, salt, beans, and lemon juice in a food processor fitted with the chopping blade until fairly smooth. Scrape down the inside of the canister, then add the oil in a thin stream through the feed tube as the machine runs to create a rich spread.

Tip: If you've refrigerated the spread, let it come back to room temperature on the counter for up to 1 hour before serving for the best flavor.

¥¶ CHICKPEA HUMMUS

Make chickpea hummus using the same process as above but substitute 3 cups drained and rinsed canned chickpeas for the beans. Also add ¼ cup tahini (a sesame-seed paste) and increase the fresh lemon juice to 3 tablespoons.

¥¶ TOASTED SPICED CHICKPEAS

Yield: 1½ cups

You can even turn chickpeas into a snack! A bowl of these can be found at my house when I have friends over for happy hour or a potluck moai.

1 (15-ounce) can chickpeas, drained and rinsed (about 1¾ cups)

3 tablespoons extra-virgin olive oil
2 teaspoons ground cumin
½ teaspoon garlic salt
½ teaspoon chili powder
¼ teaspoon freshly ground black pepper

1. Position the rack in the center of the oven and heat the oven to 350°F.
2. Toss the chickpeas, oil, cumin, garlic salt, chili powder, and black pepper in a large bowl until well coated and uniform. Pour onto a large, lipped baking sheet and spread into one layer.
3. Bake until browned and crisp, stirring occasionally, 45 to 60 minutes. Set the baking sheet on a wire rack and cool for 10 minutes. Use a slotted spoon to transfer the chickpeas to a serving bowl. Serve warm or at room temperature with plenty of napkins.

¶¶ SARDINIAN-STYLE PIZZA WITH EGGPLANT

Yield: 1 serving (can be multiplied at will for additional servings)

Eggplant is a customary topping for pizza in Sardinia, and wafer-thin pane carasau makes a healthy crust. If you can't find this type of Sardinian flat bread, substitute a whole-grain English muffin for a quick lunch or breakfast for one. Just slice off a few extra pieces of eggplant when making one of the suggested Blue Zones eggplant recipes and save it to make this pizza for breakfast or lunch the next day.

2 teaspoons olive oil
2 ¼-inch-thick slices Italian eggplant
½ pane carasau, broken in half; or 1 whole-grain English muffin, lightly toasted
3 tablespoons Sardinian Tomato Sauce (page 270)
2 tablespoons finely grated pecorino Romano (about 1 ounce)
¼ teaspoon dried oregano

1. Position the rack in the center of the oven and heat to 400°F.
2. Warm the oil in a small skillet set over medium heat. Add the eggplant and cook, turning once, until soft, about 4 minutes.
3. Put the pane carasau or muffin with the cut side up on a baking sheet. Top each half with a slice of the eggplant, 1½ tablespoons of the tomato sauce, 1 tablespoon of the grated cheese, and a pinch of dried oregano. Bake until hot and bubbling, about 5 minutes. Cool a minute or two before enjoying.

¶ EGGPLANT AND ZUCCHINI CASSEROLE

<u>Yield: 2 servings</u>

This vegetarian main course features summer vegetables popular in Sardinia. It's a bit like Sardinian eggplant Parmesan! You can also serve it alongside cooked and drained whole wheat pasta tossed in a little olive oil and minced garlic.

1 medium Italian eggplant (about 12 ounces), stemmed, peeled, and sliced into ¼-inch-thick rounds

1 medium zucchini (about 5 ounces), sliced lengthwise into ¼-inch-thick strips

1 medium yellow summer squash (about 4 ounces), sliced lengthwise into ¼-inch-thick strips

1 tablespoon salt

2 tablespoons extra-virgin olive oil, plus more for the baking pan

1 medium yellow or white onion, chopped (about 1 cup)

1 small red bell pepper, stemmed, cored, and chopped (about ½ cup)

1 tablespoon minced garlic

1 (14-ounce) can diced tomatoes (about 1¾ cups)

½ cup chopped fresh basil leaves

1 tablespoon minced fresh rosemary leaves or ½ tablespoon dried ground rosemary

½ cup finely grated pecorino Romano (about 4 ounces)

1. Spread the eggplant slices, zucchini strips, and squash strips on paper towels on your work surface; sprinkle with half of the salt. Turn the vegetables and sprinkle with the remaining salt. Set aside for 30 minutes, then rinse the vegetables and pat dry with fresh paper towels.

2. Position the rack in the center of the oven and heat the oven to 400°F. Lightly oil the inside of a 9-inch square baking dish.

3. Warm the oil in a large skillet set over medium heat. Add the onion and bell pepper; cook, stirring often, until very soft but not brown, about 7 minutes. Add the garlic and cook until fragrant, about 20 seconds.

4. Stir in the tomatoes, basil, and rosemary. Bring to a simmer, then reduce the heat to low and cook, uncovered, until the consistency of a thick sauce, about 15 minutes, stirring often.

5. Spread half the tomato sauce in the bottom of the prepared baking dish. Top with even layers of the eggplant rounds, zucchini strips, and summer squash strips in that order. Spread the remaining tomato sauce on top and sprinkle with the grated cheese.

6. Bake until bubbly and lightly browned, about 45 minutes. Cool on a wire rack for 10 minutes before serving.

¶¶ MACARONI WITH FRESH TOMATO AND BASIL SAUCE

Yield: 4 servings

This is a tasty and quick summer meal you can find in both Sardinia and Ikaria.

2 tablespoons extra-virgin olive oil
4 large red globe, beefsteak, or red heirloom tomatoes, chopped (about 3 cups)
2 tablespoons chopped fresh basil leaves
1 tablespoon minced garlic
½ teaspoon salt
¼ teaspoon freshly ground black pepper
8 ounces whole wheat durum semolina macaroni, cooked and drained according to the package instructions
½ cup finely grated pecorino Romano (about 4 ounces)

1. Warm the oil in a large saucepan set over medium heat. Add the tomatoes, basil, garlic, salt, and pepper. Cook, stirring often and crushing the tomatoes against the side of the saucepan with the back of a wooden spoon, until the tomatoes break down into a thickened sauce, about 15 minutes.
2. Stir in the macaroni and cheese. Serve hot.

Tip: For a more elegant presentation, place the cooked and drained pasta on a serving platter, then top with the sauce and the cheese.

¶¶ ANGEL HAIR WITH WALNUT AND FENNEL FROND PESTO

Yield: 6 servings as a first course or 4 as a main course

You can use any type of pasta shape, but to make it totally Blue Zones, be sure to use pasta made of 100 percent whole wheat. If you are sticking to a gluten-free diet, you can also find pasta made from brown rice or quinoa.

2 small fennel bulbs with stems and fronds (about 10 ounces total weight)
¼ cup chopped walnuts
1 tablespoon minced garlic
½ teaspoon salt
⅓ cup plus 1 tablespoon extra-virgin olive oil
1 pound whole wheat durum semolina angel hair pasta, cooked and drained according to the package instructions, ¼ cup cooking water reserved

3 tablespoons shredded pecorino Romano (about 1½ ounces)

1. Roughly chop the fennel stems and fronds (reserve the bulbs); place them in a large food processor fitted with the chopping blade. Add the walnuts, garlic, and salt. Cover and pulse, drizzling in the ⅓ cup olive oil through the feed tube, until a thick, somewhat pasty sauce.
2. If there are blemished marks on the fennel bulbs, trim these off. Quarter the bulbs and slice into thin strips. Measure out 1 cup of these slices. Reserve the remainder in a sealed plastic bag, set in the refrigerator for another use (like a fresh salad).
3. Warm the remaining 1 tablespoon olive oil in a very large skillet set over medium-high heat. Add the sliced fennel and cook, stirring frequently, until barely wilted, about 1 minute. Add the pasta; scrape in the prepared walnut sauce. Stir until well combined and heated through, about 1 minute, adding a little of the reserved pasta cooking liquid if the dish is dry (but do not make it soupy). Divide onto six plates, top each with ½ tablespoon grated cheese, and serve.

Tip: You'll most often find small fennel bulbs with tall stalks and their fronds at farmers markets or near the lettuces in large supermarkets.

¶ FAVATA

Yield: 6 servings

This recipe for pork and fennel stew is traditionally made with pork ribs and sausage, but I substituted pork tenderloin to cut the fat and calories.

1½ pounds dried, peeled fava beans
2 tablespoons extra-virgin olive oil
1 pound pork tenderloin, cut into ½-inch cubes
4 cups (1 quart) vegetable broth
1 small green cabbage, cored and coarsely chopped (about 3 cups)
3 large red ripe globe, beefsteak, or heirloom tomatoes, coarsely chopped (about 2¼ cups)
3 small fennel bulbs, trimmed and chopped (about 2 cups)
2 medium yellow or white onions, coarsely chopped (about 2 cups)
2 tablespoons loosely packed fresh Italian flat-leaf parsley leaves, finely chopped
2 tablespoons loosely packed fresh mint leaves, finely chopped
½ teaspoon salt
½ teaspoon freshly ground black pepper
6 tablespoons finely grated pecorino Romano (about 3 ounces)

1. Soak the beans in a large bowl of water at room temperature for at least 10 hours but no more than 16 hours (that is, overnight). Drain in a colander set in the sink and rinse well.
2. Warm the oil in a large pot or Dutch oven set over medium heat. Add the pork and brown well, turning occasionally, about 5 minutes.
3. Pour in the broth; stir in the soaked beans, cabbage, tomatoes, fennel, onions, parsley, mint, salt, and pepper. Raise the heat to medium-high and bring to boil. Reduce the heat to low, cover, and simmer slowly, stirring often, until the favas are tender, about 45 minutes.
4. To serve, divide among six bowls and sprinkle each with 1 tablespoon grated cheese.

Tip: Make this dish in a slow cooker. Brown the pork in warmed oil in a large skillet set over medium heat for about 5 minutes. Transfer to a 5- to 6-quart slow cooker. Add all the remaining ingredients except the cheese. Stir and cook on low for 8 hours. Sprinkle with cheese to serve.

Tip: Dried fava beans are available with or without their skins. If you can only find unpeeled dried favas, you'll need to pinch off their spongy skins after soaking.

¶¶ PANE FRATTAU

Yield: 4 servings

This new-classic recipe contains four ingredients that can always be found in Sardinian homes: eggs, tomato sauce, pecorino Romano, and pane carasau, the signature bread of Sardinia. The crisp, wafer-thin pane carasau is run through broth to soften it, transforming its cracker-like texture into something reminiscent of cooked pasta. If you're fast enough, you can assemble the dish while the eggs poach. It is kind of like a Sardinian eggs Benedict, but a lot healthier!

2 cups vegetable broth
1¼ cups Sardinian Tomato Sauce (page 270)
4 sheets pane carasau or large whole wheat flat breads, broken into quarters (for a total of 16 pieces)
¾ cup finely grated pecorino Romano (about 6 ounces)
4 large eggs
1 teaspoon salt
1 teaspoon freshly ground black pepper
½ cup chopped fresh basil leaves (optional)

1. Pour the broth into a shallow pan large enough to hold a single piece of pane carasau or flat bread; warm over medium-low heat. At the same time, bring the tomato sauce to a simmer in small saucepan set over medium heat. Also fill a Dutch oven with 4 inches of water and bring to a simmer over high heat. Have 4 plates lined up on your work surface for assembly.
2. Grasp a piece of pane carasau or a quarter of the flat bread with kitchen tongs, run it through the warmed broth, and place it on a serving plate. Repeat with 3 more pieces of pane carasau or flat bread, one for each additional plate. Top each piece of bread with 1½ tablespoons tomato sauce and 1 tablespoon grated cheese. Continue in the same fashion—softened bread, sauce, and cheese—to make three layers. Then top each with a slice of softened flat bread.
3. Reduce the heat under the Dutch oven to very low. Break an egg into a small custard cup or ramekin; slip it into the liquid. Repeat with the remaining eggs, separating them as much as possible in the pot. Turn off the heat, cover, and set aside for 3 minutes, until whites are set but the yolks are runny. (Increase the steeping time to 5 minutes for firmer yolks.) Scoop up and drain each egg with a slotted spoon before setting it on top of each stack. Sprinkle each egg with ¼ teaspoon salt and black pepper. Top with basil, if desired, before serving.

Tip: To remove as much water as possible from the poached eggs, blot the bottom of the slotted spoon with paper towels before transferring the egg to the stack.

ROASTED SARDINES

<u>Yield: 4 servings</u>

It's still up for debate as to what came first: the name of the island or these little swimmers that inhabit its waters. Whichever, sardines are abundant in Sardinia and people all over the island cook them by the hundreds. The payback is an abundance of heart-protecting omega-3 fatty acids. Sardines are a top source of these fatty acids, second only to herring. Depending on where you live, fresh sardines may not be all that easy to come by; but you should be able to find them in Italian or Asian markets, or your fishmonger should be able to get them for you on request. Ordering them online is another option. Makes sure the sardines are scaled for you. For a big weekend lunch, serve this dish with Melis Family Minestrone (page 265) and Horta (page 246).

½ cup extra-virgin olive oil
1 pound fresh sardines, gutted and scaled
½ cup loosely packed fresh Italian flat-leaf parsley leaves, chopped
4 garlic cloves, peeled and slivered

¼ teaspoon salt, preferably sea salt
¼ cup dry white wine such as pinot gris
Lemon wedges, for garnish

1. Position the rack in the center of the oven and heat the oven to 400°F.
2. Pour ¼ cup of the olive oil into a 9 x 13-inch baking pan; tip the pan to coat evenly and thoroughly. Lay the sardines in a single layer, just far enough apart so they do not touch. Sprinkle with the parsley, garlic, and salt. Drizzle the remaining ¼ cup of olive oil over the sardines.
3. Bake for 5 minutes. Pour the wine over the sardines and continue baking until the fish flakes when pricked with a fork, about 5 minutes longer. Cool in their baking dish on a wire rack for 5 minutes before serving. Offer lemon wedges for squeezing the juice over the fish.

Tip: Most sardines sold in the United States are already gutted and scaled. But if not, ask the fishmonger to do it for you (and remove the heads if you're squeamish). Or look for frozen gutted and scaled sardines in the freezer case at high-end supermarkets; unpack from the box and thaw in a large bowl set in the refrigerator for 24 to 36 hours.

ROTELLE WITH CHOPPED PORK AND TOMATO

Yield: 4 servings

After peasants butcher a pig, cut up the meat, and make their sausages, there are always bits and pieces of meat left over. Because nothing goes to waste, these scraps are gathered up and made into a pork-tomato sauce that is served over pasta. Here we use lean ground pork to cut back on the fat a bit. If you can't find lean ground pork at your supermarket, see the tip below on making your own at home.

8 ounces lean ground pork
1 tablespoon minced garlic
1 teaspoon red wine vinegar
3 tablespoons extra-virgin olive oil
1 medium yellow or white onion, chopped (about 1 cup)
1½ cups Sardinian Tomato Sauce (page 270) or jarred plain marinara sauce
1 large ripe red globe, beefsteak, or heirloom tomato, chopped (about ¾ cup)
½ pound rotelle or other spiral-shaped pasta, cooked and drained according to the package directions, ¼ cup cooking water reserved
½ cup finely grated pecorino Romano (about 4 ounces)

1. Put the pork in a large bowl; stir in the garlic and vinegar until coated. Cover and refrigerate for 2 hours.
2. Warm 1 tablespoon of the oil in a large skillet set over medium heat. Add the onion and cook, stirring often, until translucent, about 3 minutes. Add the pork and brown well, stirring to break it up, about 5 minutes.
3. Add the tomato or marinara sauce and the fresh tomato. Continue cooking, stirring occasionally and breaking up the tomato chunks with the back of a wooden spoon, until thick and bubbling, about 5 minutes.
4. Add the rotelle and a little of the reserved cooking water to help break up the pasta. Add more water if the skillet seems dry. Cook until hot, stirring often, about 1 minute. Pour onto a large serving platter or individual plates; top with the remaining 2 tablespoons of olive oil and the grated cheese.

Tip: If you can't find lean ground pork, buy ½ pound center-cut boneless pork loin or center-cut boneless pork loin chops. Slice into ½-inch-thick rounds, then cut these into ½-inch pieces. Place in a large food processor fitted with the chopping blade; pulse until coarsely ground.

ADVENTIST RECIPES

¶¶ SLOW-COOKER OATMEAL

<u>Makes 4 servings</u>

Oatmeal is a favorite breakfast among Seventh-day Adventists. It's one of mine too. Here's an Adventist-inspired way to make your morning oatmeal an instant success. Always use steel-cut oats, never quick-cooking or even regular rolled oats. Stir your breakfast in the slow cooker the night before and have it wait-ing for you when you wake up in the morning. Any extra will keep in a sealed container in the refrigerator for up to 4 days. Loosen it up with a little soy milk when reheating in a microwave.

1½ cups steel-cut oats
½ teaspoon salt

Stir the oats, salt, and 6 cups water in a 5- to 6-quart slow cooker. Cover and cook on low for 6 hours. The mixture can stay covered and on the keep-warm setting for up to 2 hours.

Tip: For more flavor, use 3 cups water and 3 cups soy milk to cook the oats.

Tip: Fill your bowl and kick up the flavor by adding one or more of the following: ground cinnamon, grated nutmeg, chopped toasted nuts, minced peeled fresh ginger, maple syrup, honey, agave nectar, shredded coconut, raisins, chopped dried apples, chopped pitted dates, sliced bananas, blueberries, and/ or blackberries.

¶| HOMEMADE GRANOLA

Yield: About 6 cups or 12 servings

Seventh-day Adventists believe breakfast is the most important meal of the day. One of the ways they like to start their day is with a bowl of granola. It's often made with cholesterol-lowering oats. To make it a totally Blue Zones breakfast, serve it with goat's or soy milk. This homemade granola will keep in a sealed, airtight container for about 2 months.

3 cups rolled oats (do not use quick-cooking or steel-cut oats)
½ cup chopped unsalted nuts, such as walnuts, pecans, and/or almonds
⅓ cup honey
¼ cup walnut oil, pecan oil, or olive oil
2 teaspoons vanilla extract
½ teaspoon ground cinnamon
½ teaspoon grated nutmeg
¼ teaspoon salt
½ cup dried berries or other chopped dried fruit, such as apples, pears, or pitted dates

1. Position the rack in the center of the oven and heat the oven to 350°F.
2. Mix the oats, nuts, honey, oil, vanilla, cinnamon, nutmeg, and salt in a large bowl until well combined. Spread onto a large lipped baking sheet.
3. Bake for 10 minutes. Stir and continue baking until golden brown, about another 10 minutes. Place the baking sheet on a wire rack. Sprinkle the dried berries or fruit on top; stir well. Cool to room temperature, about 1 hour.

Tip: For a bigger pop of flavor, use a nut oil to match the nut you've chosen: pecan oil with pecans or almond oil with almonds. Nut oils should be refrigerated once opened—and will stay fresh for about 2 months. In a pinch, substitute canola oil.

Tip: Vary the granola by decreasing the rolled oats to 2 cups and adding 1 cup rolled barley flakes.

¶ BLUE ZONES SMOOTHIE

<u>Yield: 2 servings (can be doubled)</u>

I developed this smoothie while working on the Albert Lea Project and served it to 300 people during a breakfast one Fourth of July. It all disappeared.

1 cup frozen blueberries (do not thaw)
1 cup unsweetened almond milk
½ tablespoon honey
¼ teaspoon vanilla extract
⅛ teaspoon ground cinnamon
⅛ teaspoon salt, optional

Place all the ingredients in a blender. Cover and blend until smooth and creamy. Divide between two glasses to serve.

Tip: Substitute the unsweetened almond milk for 1 cup unsweetened soy or coconut milk.

¶ TLT ON TOAST

<u>Yield: 4 servings</u>

TLT—tofu, lettuce, and tomato—is a vegetarian take on the traditional BLT. This dish is inspired by the Loma Linda University School of Medicine Alumni Association's An Apple A Day *cookbook.*

12 ounces firm tofu
1 tablespoon sesame, peanut, or extra-virgin olive oil
1 tablespoon soy sauce
4 slices sourdough or whole-grain bread, toasted
4 tomato slices
1 cup shredded lettuce, such as iceberg or romaine

1. Wrap the tofu block in a paper towel and gently squeeze out any excess moisture over the sink. You may also place the wrapped tofu block on a shallow plate and then top with a plate and a weight, such as a large can of vegetables; set aside for 10 minutes. Unwrap and cut the tofu lengthwise into 4 equal pieces.
2. Warm the oil in a medium skillet set over medium heat. Add the tofu pieces and cook for 2 minutes. Sprinkle with half the soy sauce and turn. Continue

cooking until lightly browned, about 2 more minutes. Sprinkle with the remaining soy sauce.

3. Transfer each piece of tofu to a piece of toast. Top each with a tomato slice and ¼ cup shredded lettuce. Serve open-faced.

Tip: As a spread in place of the traditional mayonnaise, try some ripe, peeled, and pitted avocado mashed with a little lime or lemon juice. Yum!

Tip: Skip the skillet entirely and substitute sliced avocado for the tofu to make an ALT: avocado, lettuce, and tomato.

¶¶ MARINATED ANTIPASTO

Yield: 10 servings

A simple crudités (raw vegetables) platter that can be found at Seventh-day Adventist church socials. So here's enough for crowds! I like to put it out for happy hour. You can also make it part of a lunch or feature it for dinner.

¾ cup extra-virgin olive oil
¼ cup balsamic vinegar
1 teaspoon minced garlic
1 teaspoon finely chopped fresh marjoram leaves
½ teaspoon salt
4 large red, yellow, green, and/or orange bell peppers, stemmed, cored, and cut into 1-inch slices
8 ounces small broccoli florets (about 2 cups)
8 ounces small cauliflower florets (about 2 cups)
8 ounces white or cremini mushrooms, halved (about 2 cups)
1 (15-ounce) can baby corn on the cob, drained and rinsed (about 2 cups)
15 medium scallions, trimmed and cut into 3-inch lengths
1 pound cherry or grape tomatoes (about 3 cups)
2 (6-ounce) jars marinated artichoke hearts, drained and halved (about 2 cups)
12 ounces shelled walnuts (about 2 cups)
8 ounces pitted black olives (about 1 cup)
2 tablespoons finely chopped fresh oregano leaves or fresh basil leaves

1. Whisk the olive oil, vinegar, garlic, marjoram, and salt in a very large bowl, large container, or even a Dutch oven until well combined. Add the bell peppers, broccoli, cauliflower, mushrooms, baby corn, and scallions. Toss well until the vegetables are thoroughly coated in the dressing. Cover with plastic wrap or

a tight-fitting lid and refrigerate for at least 8 hours or up to 24 hours, tossing the vegetables a couple of times as they marinate.
2. Arrange the marinated vegetables on a large platter. Scatter the tomatoes, artichoke hearts, walnuts, and olives on the vegetables and around the platter. Sprinkle with oregano or basil to serve.

Tip: Slice larger broccoli and cauliflower florets into bite-size bits.

QUINOA SALAD WITH SWEET POTATOES AND PEARS

<u>Yield: 4 servings</u>

This salad is a meal in one bowl. It features lots of foods popular with Adventists and also in other Blue Zones. Serve it for lunch or dinner.

¼ cup extra-virgin olive oil
¾ cup uncooked white or red quinoa
1 large sweet potato (about 12 ounces), peeled and cut into ½-inch cubes
2 tablespoons balsamic vinegar
½ teaspoon salt
¼ teaspoon freshly ground black pepper
6 cups arugula, preferably baby arugula
2 medium red-skinned pears, cored and thinly sliced
½ medium red onion, sliced into thin half-moons
½ cup packed fresh Italian flat-leaf parsley leaves, roughly chopped
¼ cup packed fresh mint leaves, preferably spearmint leaves, roughly chopped

1. Position the rack in the center of the oven and heat the oven to 400°F.
2. Warm 1 tablespoon of the oil in a medium saucepan set over medium heat. Add the quinoa and cook, stirring often, until lightly toasted, about 2 minutes. Pour in 1½ cups water, raise the heat to high, and bring to a boil. Cover, reduce the heat to low, and simmer slowly until the water has been absorbed, about 15 minutes. Remove from the heat and set aside, covered, for 10 minutes. Fluff with a fork, spread on a large plate, and refrigerate for at least 30 minutes or up to 4 hours.
3. Toss the sweet potato cubes with 1 tablespoon of the olive oil on a large rimmed baking sheet. Bake until golden brown, stirring once, about 30 minutes. Cool on the baking sheet for 20 to 30 minutes.
4. Whisk the remaining 2 tablespoons of oil with the vinegar, salt, and pepper in a large salad bowl. Add the arugula, pears, onion, parsley, and mint, as well as the chilled quinoa and sweet potatoes. Toss gently but well to serve.

¶¶ EASY TOMATO SALSA

Yield: About 2 cups

Let this salsa stand for about an hour to intensify the flavors. But do so at room temperature, because refrigeration robs tomatoes of some of their flavor. If you don't feel you're going to use this much, feel free to cut the recipe in half. If your tomatoes have been refrigerated, let them come back to room temperature to bring back some, if not all, of their ripe richness. Serve with whole-grain flat bread for dipping or spooned over grilled fish fillets, scrambled eggs, or opened, hot, baked potatoes.

2 medium red globe, beefsteak, or heirloom tomatoes (about 8 ounces each), chopped
1 small red onion, finely diced (about ½ cup)
¼ cup finely chopped fresh cilantro leaves
2 tablespoons red wine vinegar
1 tablespoon fresh lime juice
1 teaspoon minced garlic
½ teaspoon salt
¼ teaspoon freshly ground black pepper

1. Stir the tomatoes, onion, cilantro, vinegar, lime juice, and garlic in a medium bowl and set aside at room temperature for 1 hour.
2. Stir in the salt and pepper just before serving.

¶¶ AVOCADO SALSA

Yield: About 4 cups

The vegetarian foods made by Seventh-day Adventists are heavily influenced by Mexican cuisine. With avocados ubiquitous in southern California, this condiment is popular as a side dish or topping to vegetarian burgers, loaves, and fish dishes.

⅓ cup extra-virgin olive oil
¼ cup fresh lemon juice
1 tablespoon fresh lime juice
½ teaspoon dried oregano
½ teaspoon salt
½ teaspoon freshly ground black pepper
4 ripe Hass avocados, halved, pitted, peeled, and chopped
1½ cups frozen corn kernels, thawed, or fresh kernels cut off the cob
1 medium red bell pepper, stemmed, cored, and chopped (about 1 cup)
1 small red onion, chopped (about ¾ cup)

½ cup sliced pitted black olives, preferably Kalamata olives
Up to 2 tablespoons minced garlic

1. Whisk the olive oil, lemon juice, lime juice, oregano, salt, and pepper in a large bowl until well combined. Add the avocados and toss gently to keep them from browning.
2. Add the corn, bell pepper, onion, and olives. Toss gently. Cover and chill for at least 4 hours or up to 8 hours before serving.

Tip: For a more sour flavor, substitute cider vinegar for the lemon juice.

¶¶ STUFFED ACORN SQUASH

<u>Yield: 4 servings</u>

Quinoa is one whole grain that's getting more and more well known. And no wonder! Ounce for ounce, it packs a bigger protein punch than most other whole grains. Serve with a large green salad and you have all your bases covered—fruit, vegetable, grain, fiber, greens, protein, and complex carbohydrates. If blood oranges aren't available in your area, use tangerines.

4 large acorn squash (about 1 pound each), stemmed, halved, and seeded
1 tablespoon extra-virgin olive oil, plus more for the baking sheet
6 medium scallions, trimmed and thinly sliced
1 small celery stalk, diced (about 3 tablespoons)
½ cup dried cranberries, blueberries, currants, or raisins
½ cup chopped walnuts
⅓ cup dried apricots, soaked in warm water for 15 minutes, drained, and diced
1 teaspoon dried sage
1 cup uncooked long-grain brown rice, such as brown basmati, cooked and drained without salt but according to package directions (about 2 cups cooked rice)
1 cup white or red quinoa, cooked and drained without salt but according to package directions (about 1½ cups cooked quinoa)
½ cup fresh blood orange juice
½ teaspoon salt, preferably sea salt
½ teaspoon freshly ground black pepper

1. Position the rack in the center of the oven and heat the oven to 350°F. Lightly oil a large, lipped baking sheet.
2. Place the squash with the cut side down on the prepared baking sheet. Bake until tender, 30 to 40 minutes.

3. Meanwhile, warm the oil in a large skillet set over medium heat. Add the scallions and celery; cook, stirring often, until softened but not browned, about 3 minutes. Add the dried berries, nuts, dried apricots, and sage. Cook, stirring constantly, until warmed through, about 2 minutes.

4. Add the rice, quinoa, blood orange juice, salt, and pepper. Continue cooking, stirring often, until hot, about 2 minutes. Cover and set aside off the heat to keep warm.

5. Transfer the cooked squash on their baking sheet to a wire rack and cool for 5 minutes. Flip the squash over and transfer to a serving platter. Stuff the skillet mixture into the squash to serve.

¶¶ VEGETARIAN STUFFED BELLS

<u>Yield: 6 servings</u>

Brown rice and beans take the place of white rice and beef in this traditional homestyle recipe. This is especially attractive when you combine different colored bell peppers.

6 large red, green, yellow, or orange bell peppers
1 tablespoon extra-virgin olive oil
1 medium yellow or white onion, chopped (about 1 cup)
1 cup long-grain brown rice, such as brown basmati, cooked and drained without salt but according to the package directions (about 2 cups cooked rice)
2 plum tomatoes, such as Roma tomatoes, chopped
1 cup fresh corn kernels cut off the cob or frozen kernels, thawed
⅓ cup drained and rinsed canned red kidney beans
⅓ cup drained and rinsed canned black beans
¼ cup chopped pitted black olives, preferably Kalamata olives
1 tablespoon minced garlic
1 teaspoon dried oregano
1 teaspoon dried basil
2 cups Sardinian Tomato Sauce (page 270) or 2 cups plain marinara sauce
6 tablespoons finely grated pecorino Romano (about 3 ounces)

1. Slice the stem and the very tops off the peppers. Remove and discard the seeds and inner membranes with a small spoon without breaking through the flesh.

2. Warm the oil in a small skillet set over medium heat. Add the onion and cook, stirring often, until softened but not browned, about 2 minutes. Transfer to a large bowl; cool for 5 minutes.

3. Stir in the rice, tomatoes, corn, kidney beans, black beans, olives, garlic, oregano, and basil until well combined. Loosely pack into the prepared peppers.
4. Pour 1 cup of the tomato or marinara sauce in a large pot or Dutch oven; stir in ½ cup water. Set the peppers stuffing side up in the pot, side by side but not too tight. Pour the remaining tomato or marinara sauce over the peppers; top each with 1 tablespoon of the cheese.
5. Set the pot over medium-high heat and bring to a simmer. Cover tightly, reduce the heat to low, and simmer slowly until the peppers are tender, about 45 minutes. Cool for 5 minutes before serving in bowls with the sauce in the pot spooned around the peppers.

Tip: To make this dish in a 5- to 6-quart slow cooker, stuff the peppers, set them in the cooker, pour the sauce around and on top of them, and sprinkle each with 1 tablespoon of the cheese. Cover and cook on low for 6 hours. The dish can stay on the keep-warm setting, covered, for up to 3 hours.

RECIPES FROM NICOYA

▼ CREAMY SQUASH AND BEAN SOUP

Yield: 8 servings

This recipe features two of the three traditional foods of Mesoamerica: beans and squash. Corn would be the third, so eat this soup with corn tortillas. Feel free to add Easy Tomato Salsa (page 284) or bottled hot sauce.

1 pound dried white beans, such as great northern or cannellini
2 tablespoons extra-virgin olive oil
2 pounds blue Hubbard, buttercup, or butternut squash, peeled, halved, seeded, and cut into ½-inch pieces
2 cups soy milk
1 teaspoon salt
½ teaspoon freshly ground black pepper

1. Soak the beans in a big bowl of water at room temperature for at least 8 hours or up to 16 hours (that is, overnight). Drain in a colander set in the sink.
2. Warm the oil in a large pot or Dutch oven set over medium heat. Add the squash pieces and cook, stirring often, until they begin to brown at the edges, about 10 minutes. Add the beans and enough water just to cover the vegetables. Bring

to a boil over high heat. Cover, reduce the heat to low, and simmer slowly until the beans and squash are tender, about 1 hour.

3. Use an immersion blender to puree the mixture in the pot. Stir in the soy milk, salt, and pepper. Stir over low heat until warmed through, about 1 minute. Serve hot.

Tip: If you don't have an immersion blender, puree the soup in batches in a food processor fitted with the chopping blade.

ψ{ TROPICAL CABBAGE SALAD

Yield: 4 servings

When Costa Ricans make a salad, they don't reach for lettuce: It's fragile and wilts in the heat. Instead, they go for hardy and long-lasting cabbage. This salad is found just about everywhere in Costa Rica. It is a mainstay of cosado, a common daily main meal that also includes beans and rice, a fried plantain, a tortilla, and a little piece of meat or an egg. It is never laden with the heavy, high-fat salad dressings we're used to seeing or the mayonnaise we put in cole slaw, the American version of cabbage salad. It is traditionally mixed with but one ingredient: lime juice.

4 cups cored and shredded green cabbage (about half a large head)
4 plum tomatoes, such as Roma tomatoes, diced (about 1 cup)
2 medium carrots, peeled and shredded through the large holes of a box grater
1 large red bell pepper, stemmed, cored, and diced (about 1 cup)
⅓ cup finely chopped fresh cilantro leaves
½ cup fresh lime juice
½ teaspoon salt

1. Mix the cabbage, tomatoes, carrot, bell pepper, and cilantro in a large serving bowl. The salad can be made to this point; cover and refrigerate for up to 4 hours.
2. Add the lime juice and salt. Toss well to serve.

ψ{ GAZPACHO

Yield: 6 servings

This Nicoyan interpretation of the Spanish staple is full of vegetables found in Costa Rican gardens. A one-cup serving is equal to two servings of vegetables.

2½ pounds red globe, beefsteak, or heirloom tomatoes, peeled and diced (about 5 cups)
1 large green bell pepper, stemmed, cored, and diced (about 1 cup)
1 large yellow bell pepper, stemmed, cored, and diced (about 1 cup)
6 medium scallions, trimmed and thinly sliced (about 1 cup)
½ cup plain tomato juice, or more as necessary
¼ cup fresh lime juice or red wine vinegar
1 tablespoon tomato paste
1 teaspoon minced garlic
½ teaspoon salt
¼ teaspoon freshly ground black pepper
¼ teaspoon ground dried cayenne or bottled hot red pepper sauce
Finely chopped fresh cilantro leaves, for garnish
Finely chopped fresh Italian flat-leaf parsley leaves, for garnish
Lime wedges, for garnish

1. Place the tomatoes, bell peppers, scallions, ½ cup tomato juice, lime juice or vinegar, tomato paste, garlic, salt, pepper, and cayenne or hot red pepper sauce in a large bowl. Stir until the tomato paste dissolves and everything is well blended.
2. Ladle half the mixture into a food processor fitted with the chopping blade or a large blender. Cover and process or blend until fairly smooth, less than 1 minute. Pour back into the bowl and stir well.
3. Cover and refrigerate for at least 2 hours or up to 2 days. Stir in additional tomato juice if the soup becomes too thick. Ladle into bowls and garnish each with cilantro, parsley, and lime wedges.

Tip: To peel tomatoes, drop them in boiling water until the skins crack, about 1 minute. Transfer to a bowl of ice water and cool to room temperature, then slip off the skins with your fingers. Or buy a serrated tomato peeler, available at many cookware stores and their online outlets.

¶¶ PLANTAINS TWO WAYS

In Nicoya the local banana, the cuadrado, *is a staple. Like the more common plantain, it is used in both its green and ripe states. The cooked green fruit is more savory and starchy, while the cooked ripe fruit is sweet. Plantains are available in most supermarkets; green plantains are bright green while ripe plantains are yellow with many black streaks and spots. Here are two recipes to use to get to know plantains. It's easy to make Plantains Patacones Style to go with your gallo pinto. Enjoy Sweet Plantains with a meal or for dessert.*

¶ PLANTAINS PATACONES STYLE

Yield: 4 to 6 servings

2 green (or unripe) plantains
3 tablespoons canola oil

1. Use a paring knife to peel the plantains. Slice the fruit crosswise into ½-inch-thick rounds.
2. Warm 2 tablespoons of the oil in a large skillet set over medium heat. Add the plantains in a single layer and cook, until they just start to brown, about 6 minutes, turning once.
3. Put cooked plantain slices on a paper towel–lined cutting board. Gently smash each slice with the flat bottom of a sturdy glass or heavy saucepan until they're about ¼-inch thick. The slices may be cracked but should hold together.
4. Return the skillet to medium heat; add the remaining 1 tablespoon of oil. Add the flattened plantain slices and cook until golden brown and tender, turning once, about 3 minutes. Serve hot (*patacones* tend to get tough when cold).

¶ SWEET PLANTAINS

Yield: 4 to 6 servings

2 very ripe plantains
3 tablespoons canola or coconut oil
Sea salt, for garnish (optional)
Ground cinnamon, for garnish (optional)

1. Peel the plantains. Slice the fruit crosswise into ¼-inch-thick rounds.
2. Warm the oil in a large skillet set over medium heat. Add the plantains in a single layer and cook for 1½ minutes. Turn and continue cooking until golden brown, about 1 minute.
3. Remove to a paper towel–lined plate to drain briefly—but serve hot. If desired, dust with sea salt and/or cinnamon before serving.

Tip: Ripe plantains should have lots of black streaks on the peels. In general, the blacker, the sweeter. Many people buy green plantains and ripen them at home on a banana stand.

¶ PANCHITA'S GALLO PINTO

If you ever visit Costa Rica, you won't leave the country without tasting gallo pinto—*black beans and rice. Gallo pinto is the national dish, eaten with just about everything and at every meal, even breakfast. Here are two recipes for gallo pinto. The first recipe comes straight from centenarian Panchita Castillo's kitchen.*

2 tablespoons corn, canola, or vegetable oil

1 small yellow or white onion, chopped (about ¾ cup)

2 teaspoons minced garlic

2 cups drained and rinsed canned black beans or drained and rinsed cooked black beans (page 233)

1½ cups long-grain white rice, such as white basmati, cooked and drained without salt but according to the package directions (about 3 cups cooked rice)

½ teaspoon salt

¼ teaspoon freshly ground black pepper

2 tablespoons packed fresh cilantro leaves, chopped

Up to 2 teaspoons minced and seeded habanero chili, optional

1. Warm the oil in a large saucepan set over medium heat. Add the onion and cook, stirring often, until softened, about 3 minutes. Add the garlic and cook until fragrant, about 20 seconds.
2. Pour in the beans and 1 cup water. Raise the heat to medium-high and bring to a full simmer, stirring gently to keep the beans intact. Gently stir in the rice, salt, and pepper until combined and hot, about 2 minutes. Stir in the cilantro and habanero, if desired, before serving.

Tip: Habanero chilies are incendiary devices. If you're not used to working with them, use only the smallest amount. You can always add more when you make this again. Never touch your hands to your eyes or other sensitive bits until you've rubbed them thoroughly with oil and washed them thoroughly with hot, soapy water. (The chili oil is fat soluble, not water soluble.)

¶ GALLO PINTO WITH SALSA LIZANO

Yield: 4 servings

The second recipe for gallo pinto includes the "secret" ingredient that makes Costa Rica's beans and rice taste different: Salsa Lizano, a slightly sweet and tangy condiment that is as common in Costa Rican homes and restaurants as ketchup is in North America. Among its ingredients are many Blue Zones foods, including cauliflower, onions, peppers, and turmeric. Unfortunately, Salsa Lizano isn't a common commodity in American supermarkets, but the sauce can be purchased online. Even Costa Ricans agree that another thin brown sauce very common to U.S. kitchens, Worcestershire sauce, is a fine substitute for Salsa Lizano in authentic gallo pinto.

2 tablespoons extra-virgin olive oil
1 medium yellow or white onion, diced (about 1 cup)
½ cup seeded, cored, and chopped red bell pepper (about half a large bell pepper)
1 tablespoon minced garlic
1 teaspoon ground cumin
3 tablespoons Salsa Lizano or Worcestershire sauce
2 cups drained and rinsed canned black beans or drained and rinsed cooked black beans (page 233)
1 cup long-grain white rice, such as white basmati, cooked and drained without salt but according to the package instructions (about 2 cups cooked rice)
Finely chopped fresh cilantro leaves, for garnish
Finely chopped scallions, for garnish

1. Warm the oil in a large skillet set over medium heat. Add the onion and bell pepper; cook, stirring often, until the onion is translucent, about 3 minutes. Add the garlic and cumin; cook until fragrant, about 20 seconds. Add the Salsa Lizano or Worcestershire sauce; scrape up any browned bits on the bottom of the skillet with this liquid.
2. Stir in the beans and rice; cook until heated through, about 3 minutes. Serve garnished with cilantro and scallions.

🍴 GALLO PINTO WITH AN EGG

For a Nicoyan breakfast, slide a fried egg on top of a serving of black beans and rice; sprinkle with finely chopped fresh cilantro leaves.

🍴 NIXTAMAL CORN TORTILLAS

Yield: 16 tortillas

You can make tortillas Nicoyan style. All you need is lime-treated corn flour, which is called masa harina. To make it easier, you may want a tortilla press. Both can be purchased at Latin American markets or online. You can also make tortillas by hand, but it takes practice to roll the dough thin enough. In any event,

I give directions for both. For the best results, use a well-seasoned cast-iron griddle or skillet. If you want to make it easier, you can purchase corn tortillas at almost any grocery store; just make sure the list of ingredients is short and simple, about like this recipe.

2 cups masa harina
¼ teaspoon baking soda
Wax paper, as needed

1. Whisk the masa harina and baking soda in a large bowl. Add 1½ cups warm tap water and stir until a soft dough forms. If the mixture won't form a soft ball of dough, add warm water in 1-tablespoon increments until it will. Cover with plastic wrap and set aside for 5 minutes.
2. Turn the dough out onto a clean, dry work surface. Knead gently for 1 minute. Divide it into 16 equal pieces, each about the size of a small plum.
3. To use a tortilla press, line the press with two small sheets of wax paper. Put one piece of dough between the sheets, close the press, and gently press down. Remove the dough between the wax paper sheets, then repeat with more wax paper and the remaining dough balls. To make tortillas by hand, put each dough ball between two pieces of wax paper and roll into a thin 6-inch round.
4. Set a griddle or skillet, preferably cast iron, over high heat until smoking. Remove one flattened dough ball from the wax paper and set on the griddle or in the pan. Cook for 30 seconds, flip with kitchen tongs, and cook until lightly toasted with tiny bubbles in the tortilla, about 30 more seconds. Transfer to a clean kitchen towel, wrap gently, and continue cooking more tortillas, keeping them warm as a stack in the towel. Serve warm.

Tip: Cool any unused tortilla to room temperature and store tightly wrapped in the kitchen towel in the refrigerator for up to 1 day. Reheat on a baking sheet 4 to 6 inches from a heated broiler for 10 seconds.

¶¶ BEAN AND SQUASH TORTILLAS WITH PAPAYA SALSA

<u>Yield: 6 servings</u>

Nicoyans eat tortillas at every meal, so the choice of when to eat this is all yours! For variety, substitute a mango or pineapple for the papaya in the salsa.

1 small ripe papaya, peeled, halved, seeded, and chopped (about 1 cup)
1 small red bell pepper, stemmed, cored, and diced (about ½ cup)

¼ cup finely chopped fresh cilantro leaves

3 tablespoons extra-virgin olive oil

2 tablespoons fresh lime juice

1½ cups drained and rinsed canned black or pinto beans or drained and rinsed cooked black or pinto beans (page 233)

1 medium yellow squash (about 4 ounces), chopped

1 cup corn kernels cut from the ear or frozen kernels, thawed

2 medium carrots, peeled and shredded through the large holes of a box grater

1 teaspoon ground cumin

Up to ½ teaspoon ground dried cayenne

¼ teaspoon salt

6 Nixtamal Corn Tortillas (page 292)

1. Stir the papaya, bell pepper, cilantro, 1 tablespoon of the olive oil, and the lime juice in a small bowl. The salsa can be made in advance; cover and set aside at room temperature for up to 4 hours.
2. Warm 1 tablespoon of the oil in a large skillet set over medium-high heat. Add the beans, squash, corn, carrots, cumin, cayenne, and salt. Cook, stirring often, until the squash is tender, about 5 minutes. Stir in the papaya salsa and set aside off the heat.
3. Set the oven rack 4 to 6 inches from the broiler element; heat the broiler for a few minutes. Lay the tortillas on a large, lipped baking sheet; brush them with the remaining 1 tablespoon of oil. Broil until warmed and lightly toasted, about 30 seconds.
4. Transfer the tortillas to 6 serving plates. Top each with a sixth of the bean mixture (a rounded ¾ cup) to serve.

¶ TROPICAL LENTIL STEW

Yield: 6 servings

All Costa Ricans have their own recipe for this stew. This is mine. The list of ingredients is long but the preparation is simple. If you don't have all the spices on hand, eliminate up to two. Doing so will alter the taste but the dish will still be delicious.

8 cups (2 quarts) vegetable broth

1½ cups brown, green, or black beluga lentils

2 large sweet potatoes (about 1 pound each), peeled and cut into ½-inch cubes

1 medium yellow or white onion, chopped (about 1 cup)

1 cup canned tomato sauce

2 teaspoons minced garlic

1 teaspoon ground cumin
1 teaspoon ground cinnamon
1 teaspoon dried ground ginger
½ teaspoon ground cardamom
½ teaspoon ground cloves
½ teaspoon grated nutmeg
½ teaspoon salt
½ teaspoon freshly ground black pepper
3 medium ripe bananas, peeled and cut into ½-inch-thick slices
2 cups pineapple chunks

1. Mix the broth, lentils, sweet potatoes, onion, tomato sauce, garlic, cumin, cin-namon, ginger, cardamom, cloves, nutmeg, salt, and pepper in a large pot or Dutch oven. Bring to a boil over high heat. Reduce the heat to low and simmer, uncovered, until the lentils and sweet potatoes are tender, 50 to 60 minutes.
2. Use an immersion blender to partially puree the soup, leaving its overall texture slightly chunky. Or ladle about half the soup into a large blender, cover loosely with a clean kitchen towel, and blend until smooth before stirring this puree back into the pot. Ladle into 6 serving bowls and top each with ⅓ cup of the banana slices and ⅓ cup of the pineapple chunks.

Tip: Peeled and cored pineapple chunks are available in most supermarkets' produce sections in the refrigerator case.

￦ PICADILLO WITH MANGO AND PORK

<u>Yield: 4 servings</u>

Picadillo *means "chopped," but it's also the name of a popular dish served all over Costa Rica. It always includes some type of ground meat, vegetables in season, and potatoes. This version is served over rice, but it can be prepared and on the table in the time it takes to cook the rice.*

1½ tablespoons extra-virgin olive oil
3 tablespoons sliced almonds
8 ounces lean ground pork
1 small white or yellow onion, halved and sliced into thin half-moons
1 small red-skinned potato (about 3 ounces), peeled and diced
1 tablespoon minced garlic
1 cup Easy Tomato Salsa (page 284) or purchased tomato salsa
1 teaspoon ground cinnamon

1 teaspoon ground coriander
1 teaspoon ground cumin
1 teaspoon dried oregano
1 ripe mango, peeled, pitted, and diced
2 cups long-grain white rice, cooked and drained without salt but according to
  the package directions (about 4 cups cooked rice)
Finely chopped fresh cilantro leaves, for garnish

1. Warm ½ tablespoon of the oil in a large skillet set over medium-low heat. Add
   the almonds and cook, stirring almost constantly, until lightly browned and
   aromatic, about 1 minute. Transfer to a small bowl.
2. Set that skillet over medium heat and add the remaining 1 tablespoon of oil.
   Crumble in the ground pork and cook, stirring often, until browned, about
   4 minutes. Use a slotted spoon to remove the meat and drain it on a paper
   towel–lined plate. Pour out all but 1 tablespoon of the fat from the skillet.
3. With the skillet still over medium heat, add the onion and potato. Cook, stirring
   frequently, until lightly browned, about 5 minutes. Add the garlic and cook until
   fragrant, about 20 seconds. Stir in the salsa, cinnamon, coriander, cumin, and
   oregano. Bring to a simmer. Reduce the heat to low and simmer, uncovered,
   until thick, about 5 minutes.
4. Stir in the pork and mango. Cover and cook until thick, rich, and blended, stirring occasionally, about 5 minutes. Serve over rice, topped with the toasted
   almonds and some chopped cilantro for garnish.

Tip: For more whole-grain goodness, substitute 2 cups long-grain brown rice
for the white rice, cooked and drained without salt but according to the package
instructions.

¶¶ POLLO GUISADO

Yield: 6 servings

*Many Nicoyans raise free-range (pastured) chickens. When it's time for a special
meal, it's time for* pollo guisado—*or stewed chicken. Practically every family
has its own spin on this recipe, but it always includes a whole chicken in a broth
with lots of vegetables. Potatoes are a must. Here I only use skinned breast and
thighs to keep the fat content low. I also replaced the more traditional vegetable
oil with olive oil for the added health benefits.*

1 free-range chicken breast, skinned and cut in half
2 free-range chicken thighs, skinned

¼ teaspoon salt
¼ teaspoon freshly ground black pepper
½ cup all-purpose flour, for dredging
2 tablespoons extra-virgin olive oil
1 large yellow or white onion, halved and sliced into thin half-moons
3 cups chicken broth
1 (14-ounce) can diced tomatoes (about 1¾ cups)
½ cup dry white wine, such as chardonnay
6 medium red-skinned potatoes (about 1½ pounds), peeled and chopped
3 large carrots, peeled and sliced into thin rings
1½ cups shelled fresh peas or frozen peas, thawed
1 teaspoon dried oregano
1 teaspoon ground cumin
Finely chopped fresh Italian flat-cut parsley leaves, for garnish
Lime wedges, for garnish

1. Season the chicken with salt and pepper. Spread the flour on a large plate and dredge the chicken pieces in it, coating them evenly and well but shaking off any excess flour.

2. Warm the oil in a large pot or Dutch oven set over medium heat. Add the onion and cook, stirring often, until softened, about 4 minutes. Push the onions to the sides of the pot and add the chicken pieces. Brown them on each side, turning once, about 5 minutes.

3. Add the broth, tomatoes, and wine. Stir well, raise the heat to medium-high, and bring to a full simmer, scraping up any browned bits on the inside bottom of the pot. Stir in the potatoes, carrots, peas, oregano, and cumin. Bring back to a simmer, then reduce the heat to low and simmer very slowly, uncovered, until the chicken is tender, about 40 minutes.

4. Use a slotted spoon to transfer the chicken pieces to a cutting board. Cover the soup off the heat to keep warm. Cool the chicken a few minutes, then tear the meat from the bones.

5. Divide the chicken among 6 serving bowls. Using a slotted spoon, top the chicken with the vegetables from the pot. Ladle enough broth into each bowl to cover the ingredients. Garnish with parsley and offer a lime wedge to squeeze the juice over each helping.

The Science Behind the Blue Zones Solution

GOALS

- To create a Blue Zones diet that as accurately as possible reflects what centenarians in each Blue Zone typically eat and how they prepare foods
- To ground that synthesis in the available scientific and scholarly research as well as in our observations based on hundreds of interviews

OUR METHODOLOGY

We first used several means to identify available research on eating patterns in each Blue Zone. These included searches of PubMed, JSTOR, and other research databases and examination of bibliographies in identified studies. Leading researchers and experts on the individual Blue Zones provided additional research, including some unpublished data, and observations.

For each Blue Zone, we identified and examined nutrition survey data, published and unpublished, and studies that included dietary surveys.

As possible, we charted average intakes (in grams per day) of foods and food groups. General distribution of food groups and macronutrients were determined and charted. Observational and descriptive studies were then used to interpret and amplify customary practices suggested by nutrition surveys. You can see a summary of the research for each Blue Zone in the following pages.

The next step was to synthesize the individual patterns we had observed and that were supported by the research data into one Blue Zones diet or eating pattern. This task was challenging because the research on nutritional and eating patterns varies widely in criteria, methods, definitions, information collected, population studied, reliability, and time frame. As a result, in addition to comparing the metrics and possible averages, we used descriptive, observational statements from older and recent studies and from leading researchers and our own observations. Based on these analyses, we created the Blue Zones Nutrition Guidelines and a Blue Zones Eating Pattern, which provides recommendations for daily intakes (based on 2,000 cal/day) of specific food groups and Blue Zones foods.

Finally, we also reviewed the broader scientific context for the Blue Zones diet by reviewing the medical and nutrition research related to issues of longevity, nutrition, eating patterns, evidence-based dietary guidelines, and health and chronic disease. Summaries of this research as it relates to each Blue Zone are provided in the following pages.

Acknowledgments

For brothers Steve, Nick, and Tony—my best friends and partners in exploration.

I owe first thanks to former *National Geographic* editor and writer Peter Miller. He helped shape the sprawling yard sale of my ideas into an elegant how-to narrative. He also expertly drafted chapters 7–9 (on the Blue Zones Project cities), because I didn't think I could objectively self-report my own deeds. Special thanks to Debbie Yost for her early contributions to the book. Mary Abbott Waite gets most of the credit for distilling the hundreds of dietary studies and surveys that form the academic foundations of this book. And foremost among the team of researchers who helped was the *New York Times's* Lia Miller, who endured unimaginable tedium in fact-checking. Mark Scarbrough and Bruce Weinstein did an outstanding job testing all the recipes.

Of the many experts around the world who contributed to this project, I'm indebted to Robert Kane, who first saw the potential of the Blue Zones and has helped guide me academically for more than a decade, and Blue Zones founding partners, Michel Poulain and Gianni Pes, who identified the Sardinia Blue Zone and helped validate and study the Nicoya and Ikaria Blue Zones. David McLain and Susan Welchman collaborated on the original Blue Zones story in *National Geographic*. Craig and Bradley Willcox, who did most of the longevity research in Okinawa, have generously advised me. The Adventist Health Study's Gary Fraser and Michael Orlich, along with their colleague Joan Sabaté, were also very helpful. I wish to thank the faculty of the University of Minnesota School of Public Health, including Robert Jeffery, John Finnegan, and especially clarinetist extraordinaire, Henry Blackburn. Daniel Ariely, Kathleen Vohs, Nicholas Christakis, Thomas Goetz, Thomas Hayden, Walter Willett, Dean Ornish, Neal Barnard, Mary Frasier, *I Quit Sugar* author Sarah Wilson, and especially mentor and *Body Worry* author Remar Sutton all reviewed the manuscript or contributed invaluable input.

In Finland, I thank Pekka Puska, to whom I owe the inspiration for the Blue Zones community project, and Vesa Korpelainen and his lovely daughter, Elisa, who guided me through the North Karelia Project.

Thea and Elias Parikos and Eleni Mazari on Ikaria have been my guides, cultural interpreters, hosts, and fellow all-night revelers in Ikaria since 2008. Luis Rosero-Bixby, lead researcher in finding the Nicoya Blue Zone, and Jorge Vindas continue to provide longevity updates from Costa Rica. Pat Weiland and Toby Brocklehurst have joined our team in identifying the sixth (still undisclosed—stay tuned) Blue Zone.

Walkability virtuoso Dan Burden, *Slim by Design* author Brian Wansink, obesity expert Leslie Lytle, and AARP's Nancy Perry Graham helped me design and execute the first Blue Zones Project in Albert Lea. But it has been Healthways CEO Ben Leedle's vision, courage, and knack for innovation that has been responsible for the Blue Zones Project spreading across America. He, along with his colleagues Michael Acker, Janet Calhoun, Erika Graves, Justin Smith, Katrina Worland, Ann Kent, Joel Spoonheim, Mary Lawyer, Shannon Sanders, Jennifer Furler, Jon Werger, Katherine McClure, Marty Leinwand, and Mike Ferris, has helped bring the Blue Zones Project to more than five million people in 20 cities. I'd like to thank Albert Lea's Ellen and Randy Kehr, Robert Graham, and Chad Adams; Wellmark's John Forsyth and Laura Jackson, and Iowa's governor, Terry Branstad; Lisa Santora and Susan Burden of the Beach Cities Health District; Barclay Berdan of the Texas Health Resources, and Fort Worth's magnificent mayor Betsy Price; HMSA's Mike Gold and Elisa Yadao; and Kauai's mayor "Chief" Bernard Carvalho, Beth Tokioka, Bill Arakaki, Dileep Baal, Bev

Brody, and Scott McFarland. These are some of the most extraordinary early adopters who have brought the Blue Zones Project to their communities.

At National Geographic, I thank my book editor, Lisa Thomas, who championed the idea of taking a magazine cover story and expanding it to three books; P.R. virtuoso Ann Day; my longtime friend on the Expeditions Council, Rebecca Martin, and my newest friend, Janet Goldstein, for her tremendous support. Tia Bastion, Miranda Bauer, and Noemia Strapazzon also contributed their extensive research talents.

At Blue Zones Minneapolis headquarters, I thank my business mentor, Tom Gegax, to whom I owe much of my success. Scott Meyer and Becky Malkerson have been our advisers from the very beginning. Ed McCall and John Higgins have expertly chaired the board of directors; and the office staff—Sam Skemp, Lydia Turner, Amelia Clabots, Gwen Martin—are the engine that propels us. I am also grateful to Tom Moudry, Gayle Winegar, Dean Phillips, Tom Heuer, Rob Perez, and Rudy Maxa.

And to the members of the media who have helped bring the Blue Zones message to America, I thank Mehmet Oz, who first put the Blue Zones on *Oprah* and then on his own show; CNN's Bill Weir, Sanjay Gupta, and Danielle Dellorto; and Diane Sawyer, Oprah Winfrey, Diane Reeves, and especially Patty Neger, who helped put the Blue Zones on the map a decade ago.

Finally, to *New York Times* best-selling *Veganist* author Kathy Freston, who contributed her vast dietary expertise, keen insights, and cruciferous affection to me throughout the writing of this book: You are at the center of my Blue Zone.

Selected Bibliography

IKARIA

Ikarian Study, 2009, nutrition data, unpublished. Supplied to author by lead study researcher, Dr. Christina Chrysohoou.

Panagiotakos, D. B., C. Chrysohoou, G. Siasos, K. Zisimos, J. Skoumas, C. Pitsavos, and C. Stefanadis. "Sociodemographic and Lifestyle Statistics of Oldest Old People (>80 Years) Living in Ikaria Island: The Ikaria Study." *Cardiology Research and Practice* (2011), article ID 679187.

Research on Potential Health Benefits of Ikarian Diet and Supporting Research
Antonogeorgos, G., D. B. Panagiotakos, C. Pitsavos, C. Papageorgiou, C. Chrysohoou, G. N. Papadimitriou, and C. Stefanadis. "Understanding the Role of Depression and Anxiety on Cardiovascular Disease Risk, Using Structural Equation Modeling; The Mediating Effect of the Mediterranean Diet and Physical Activity: The ATTICA Study." *Annals of Epidemiology* (September 2012), 630–37.

Chrysohoou, C., D. B. Panagiotakos, P. Aggelopoulos, C. M. Kastorini, I. Kehagia, C. Pitsavos, and C. Stefanadis. "The Mediterranean Diet Contributes to the Preservation of Left Ventricular Systolic Function and to the Long-Term Favorable Prognosis of Patients Who Have Had an Acute Coronary Event." *American Journal of Clinical Nutrition* (July 2010), 47–54.

Chrysohoou, C., C. Pitsavos, D. Panagiotakos, J. Skoumas, G. Lazaros, E. Oikonomou, N. Galiatsatos, M. Striggou, M. Xynogala, and C. Stefanadis. "Long-Term Fish Intake Preserves Kidney Function in Elderly Individuals: The Ikaria Study." *Journal of Renal Nutrition* (July 2013), e75–82.

Chrysohoou, C., J. Skoumas, C. Pitsavos, C. Masoura, G. Siasos, N. Galiatsatos, T. Psaltopoulou, et al. "Long-Term Adherence to the Mediterranean Diet Reduces the Prevalence of Hyperuricaemia in Elderly Individuals, Without Known Cardiovascular Disease: The Ikaria Study." *Maturitas* (September 2011), 58–64.

Chrysohoou, C., G. Tsitsinakis, G. Siassos, T. Psaltopoulou, N. Galiatsatos, V. Metaxa, G. Lazaros, et al. "Fish Consumption Moderates Depressive Symptomatology in Elderly Men and Women from the IKARIA Study." *Cardiology Research and Practice* (2011), article ID 219578.

Covas, M. I., V. Konstantinidou, and M. Fitó. "Olive Oil and Cardiovascular Health." *Journal of Cardiovascular Pharmacology* (December 2009), 477–82.

Kavouras, S. A., D. B. Panagiotakos, C. Pitsavos, C. Chrysohoou, G. Arnaoutis, Y. Skoumas, and C. Stefanadis. "Physical Activity and Adherence to Mediterranean Diet Increase Total Antioxidant Capacity: The ATTICA Study." *Cardiology Research and Practice* (2011), article ID 248626.

Lasa, A., J. Miranda, M. Bulló, R. Casas, J. Salas-Salvadó, I. Larretxi, R. Estruch, V. Ruiz-Gutiérrez, and M. P. Portillo. "Comparative Effect of Two Mediterranean Diets Versus a Low-Fat Diet on Glycaemic Control in Individuals With Type 2 Diabetes." *European Journal of Clinical Nutrition* (Epub February 12, 2014) [ahead of print].

Martín-Peláez, S., M. I. Covas, M. Fitó, A. Kušar, and I. Pravst. "Health Effects of Olive Oil Polyphenols: Recent Advances and Possibilities for the Use of Health Claims." *Molecular Nutrition and Food Research* (May 2013), 760–71.

Naska, A., E. Oikonomou, A. Trichopoulou, T. Psaltopoulou, and D. Trichopoulos. "Siesta in Healthy Adults and Coronary Mortality in the General Population." *Archives of Internal Medicine* (February 12, 2007), 296–301.

Oikonomou, E., C. Chrysohoou, D. Tsiachris, G. Vogiatzi, E. Gialafos, G. Marinos, G. Tsitsinakis, et al. "Gender Variation of Exercise-Induced Anti-Arrhythmic Protection: The Ikaria Study." *QJM* (December 2011), 1035–43.

Pryde, M. M., and W. B. Kannel. "Efficacy of Dietary Behavior Modification for Preserving Cardiovascular Health and Longevity." *Cardiology Research and Practice* (2011), article ID 820457.

Siasos, G., C. Chrysohoou, D. Tousoulis, E. Oikonomou, D. Panagiotakos, M. Zaromitidou, K. Zisimos, et al. "The Impact of Physical Activity on Endothelial Function in Middle-Aged and Elderly Subjects: The Ikaria Study." *Hellenic Journal of Cardiology* (March–April 2013), 94–101.

Siasos, G., E. Oikonomou, C. Chrysohoou, D. Tousoulis, D. Panagiotakos, M. Zaromitidou, K. Zisimos, et al. "Consumption of a Boiled Greek Type of Coffee Is Associated With Improved Endothelial Function: The Ikaria Study." *Vascular Medicine* (April 2013), 55–62.

Sofi, F., C. Macchi, R. Abbate, G. F. Gensini, and A. Casini. "Mediterranean Diet and Health Status: An Updated Meta-Analysis and a Proposal for a Literature-Based Adherence Score." *Public Health Nutrition* (Epub November 29, 2013), 14 pp.

Tyrovolas, S., and D. B. Panagiotakos. "The Role of Mediterranean Type of Diet on the Development of Cancer and Cardiovascular Disease in the Elderly: A Systematic Review." *Maturitas* (February 2010), 122–30.

OKINAWA

Research Based on National Survey Data

Akisaka, M., L. Asato, Y. C. Chan, M. Suzuki, T. Uezato, and S. Uamamoto. "Energy and Nutrient Intakes of Okinawan Centenarians." *Journal of Nutritional Science and Vitaminology* (June 1996), 241–48.

Shibata, H., H. Nagai, H. Haga, S. Yasumura, T. Suzuki, and Y. Suyama. "Nutrition for the Japanese Elderly." *Nutrition and Health* (April 1992), 165–75.

Willcox, B. J., D. C. Willcox, H. Todoriki, A. Fujiyoshi, K. Yano, Q. He, J. D. Curb, and M. Suzuki. "Caloric Restriction, the Traditional Okinawan Diet, and Healthy Aging: The Diet of the World's Longest-Lived People and Its Potential Impact on Morbidity and Life Span." *Annals of the New York Academy of Sciences* (October 2007), 434–55.

Research Literature Describing Typical Foods of Traditional Okinawan Diet and Potential Benefits

Arakaki, H., and H. Sho. "Nutritional Survey on Kumejima." *The Science Bulletin of the Division of Agriculture, Home Economics & Engineering, University of the Ryukyus* (December 1962), 327–34.

Mano, R., A. Ishida, Y. Ohya, H. Todoriki, S. Takishita. "Dietary Intervention With Okinawan Vegetables Increased Circulating Endothelial Progenitor Cells in Healthy Young Women." *Atherosclerosis* (June 2009), 544–48.

Moriguchi, E. H., Y. Moriguchi, and Y. Yamori. "Impact of Diet on the Cardiovascular Risk Profile of Japanese Immigrants Living in Brazil: Contributions of the World Health Organization CARDIAC and MONALISA Studies." *Clinical and Experimental Pharmacology and Physiology* (December 2004), S5–7.

Sho, H. "History and Characteristics of Okinawan Longevity Food." *Asia Pacific Journal of Clinical Nutrition* (June 2001), 159–64.

Suzuki, M., B. J. Willcox, and D. C. Willcox. "Implications From and For Food Cultures for Cardiovascular Disease Longevity." *Asia Pacific Journal of Clinical Nutrition* (June 2001), 164–71.

Suzuki, M., D. C. Willcox, M. W. Rosenbaum, and B. J. Willcox. "Oxidative Stress and Longevity in Okinawa: An Investigation of Blood Lipid Peroxidation and Tocopherol in Okinawan Centenarians." *Current Gerontology and Geriatrics Research* (2010), article ID 380460, 10 pp.

Willcox, D. C., G. Scapagnini, and B. J. Willcox. "Healthy Aging Diets Other Than the Mediterranean: A Focus on the Okinawan Diet." *Mechanisms of Ageing and Development* (Epub January 21, 2014) [ahead of print].

Willcox, D. C., B. J. Willcox, and M. Suzuki. *The Okinawa Program: Learn the Secrets to Healthy Longevity.* Three Rivers Press, 2001.

Willcox, D. C., B. J. Willcox, H. Todoriki, and M. Suzuki. "The Okinawan Diet: Health Implications of a Low-Calorie, Nutrient-Dense, Antioxidant-Rich Dietary Pattern Low in Glycemic Load." *Journal of the American College of Nutrition* (August 2009), 500S–516S.

Yamori, Y., A. Miura, and K. Taira. "Implications From and For Food Cultures for Cardiovascular Diseases: Japanese Food, Particularly Okinawan Diets." *Asia Pacific Journal of Clinical Nutrition* (June 2001), 144–45.

Calorie Restriction and Longevity in Okinawans

Gavrilova, N. S., and L. A. Gavrilov. "Comments on Dietary Restriction, Okinawa Diet and Longevity." *Gerontology* (April 2012), 221–23.

Willcox, B. J., D. C. Willcox, H. Todoriki, K. Yano, J. D. Curb, and M. Suzuki. "Caloric Restriction, Energy Balance and Healthy Aging in Okinawans and Americans: Biomarker Differences in Septuagenarians." *Okinawan Journal of American Studies* (2007), 62–74.

Willcox, D. C., B. J. Willcox, H. Todoriki, J. D. Curb, and M. Suzuki. "Caloric Restriction and Human Longevity: What Can We Learn From the Okinawans?" *Biogerontology* (June 2006), 173–77.

Impact of Westernization on Okinawan Diet and Lifestyle

Kagawa Y. "Impact of Westernization on the Nutrition of Japanese: Changes in Physique, Cancer, Longevity and Centenarians." *Preventive Medicine* (June 1978), 205–217.

Miyagi, S., N. Iwama, T. Kawabata, and K. Hasegawa. "Longevity and Diet in Okinawa, Japan: The Past, Present and Future." *Asia-Pacific Journal of Public Health* (July 2003), S3–9.

Suzuki, M., C. Willcox, and B. Willcox. "The Historical Context of Okinawan Longevity: Influence of the United States and Mainland Japan." *Okinawan Journal of American Studies* (2007), 46–61.

Todoriki, H., D. C. Willcox, and B. J. Willcox. "The Effects of Post-War Dietary Change on Longevity and Health in Okinawa." *Okinawan Journal of American Studies* (2004), 52–61.

Physical Activity and Social Interconnection

Salen, P., and M. de Lorgeril. "The Okinawan Diet: A Modern View of an Ancestral Healthy Lifestyle." *World Review of Nutrition and Dietetics* (2011), 114–23.

Suzuki, M., M. Akisaka, I. Ashitomi, K. Higa, and H. Nozaki. "Abstract of Chronological Study Concerning ADL Among Okinawan Centenarians" [in Japanese]. *Nihon Ronen Igakkai Zasshi* (June 1995); 32:416–23.

Willcox, D. C., B. J. Willcox, S. Shimajiri, S. Kurechi, and M. Suzuki. "Aging Gracefully: A Retrospective Analysis of Functional Status in Okinawan Centenarians." *American Journal of Geriatric Psychiatry* (March 2007), 252–56.

Potential Genetic Impact on Longevity

Heilbronn, L. K., and E. Ravussin. "Calorie Restriction and Aging: Review of the Literature and Implications for Studies in Humans." *American Journal of Clinical Nutrition* (September 2003), 361–69.

Willcox, B. J., T. A. Donlon, Q. He, R. Chen, J. S. Grove, K. Yano, K. H. Masaki, D. C. Willcox, B. Rodriguez, and J. D. Curb. "FOXO3A Genotype Is Strongly Associated With Human Longevity." *Proceedings of the National Academy of Sciences of the U.S.A.* (September 16, 2008), 13987–92.

Willcox, D. C., B. J. Willcox, W.-C. Hsueh, and M. Suzuki. "Genetic Determinants of Human Longevity: Insights From the Okinawa Centenarian Study." *AGE* (December 2006), 313–32.

Selected Supporting Research for Health Benefits of Diets Similar to Okinawan Traditional Diet

Ajala, O., P. English, and J. Pinkney. "Systematic Review and Meta-Analysis of Different Dietary Approaches to the Management of Type 2 Diabetes." *American Journal of Clinical Nutrition* (March 2013), 505–16.

Khazrai, Y. M., G. Defeudis, and P. Pozzilli. "Effect of Diet on Type 2 Diabetes Mellitus: A Review." *Diabetes-Metabolism Research and Reviews* (March 2014), 24–33.

O'Keefe, J. H., N. M. Gheewala, and J. O. O'Keefe. "Dietary Strategies for Improving Post-Prandial Glucose, Lipids, Inflammation, and Cardiovascular Health." *Journal of the American College of Cardiology* (January 22, 2008), 249–55.

Rizza, W., N. Veronese, and L. Fontana. "What Are the Roles of Calorie Restriction and Diet Quality in Promoting Healthy Longevity?" *Ageing Research Reviews* (January 2014), 38–45.

Venn, B. J., and T. J. Green. "Glycemic Index and Glycemic Load: Measurement Issues and Their Effect on Diet-Disease Relationships." *European Journal of Clinical Nutrition* (December 2007), S122–31.

SARDINIA

Carbini, L. "Evoluzione del comportamento alimentare nei sardi dal secondo dopoguerra ad oggi." In *L'Uomo in Sardegna*, ed. Giovanni Floris. Zonza Editori, 1998. 153–73.

Carbini, L., T. Lantini, A. Peretti Padalino, and A. L. Scarpa. "Nutritional Surveys in Some Centers of 3 Provinces of Sardinia. II. Nutrition and Tradition" [in Italian]. *Bolletino della Società Italiana di Biologia Sperimentale* (January 30, 1981), 226–28.

Carru, C., G. M. Pes, L. Deiana, G. Baggio, C. Franceschi, D. Lio, C. R. Balistreri, G. Candore, G. Colonna-Romano, and C. Caruso. "Association Between the HFE Mutations and Longevity: A Study in Sardinian Population." *Mechanisms of Ageing and Development* (April 2003), 529–32.

Selected Bibliography

Caselli, G., and R. M. Lipsi. "Survival Differences Among the Oldest Old in Sardinia: Who, What, Where, and Why?" *Demographic Research* (March 2006), 267–94.

Caselli, G., L. Pozzi, J. W. Vaupel, L. Deiana, G. Pes, C. Carru, C. Franceschi, and G. Baggio. "Family Clustering in Sardinian Longevity: A Genealogical Approach." *Experimental Gerontology* (August 2006), 727–36.

Deiana, L., L. Ferrucci, G. M. Pes, C. Carru, G. Delitala, A. Ganau, S. Mariotti, et al. "AKEntAnnos: The Sardinia Study of Extreme Longevity." *Aging* (Milano) (June 1999), 142–49.

Franceschi, C., L. Motta, S. Valensin, R. Rapisarda, A. Franzone, M. Berardelli, M. Motta, et al. "Do Men and Women Follow Different Trajectories to Reach Extreme Longevity?" Italian Multicenter Study on Centenarians (IMUSCE)." *Aging* (Milano) (April 2000), 77–84.

Lio, D., G. M. Pes, C. Carru, F. Listì, V. Ferlazzo, G. Candore, G. Colonna-Romano, et al. "Association Between the HLA-DR Alleles and Longevity: A Study in Sardinian Population." *Experimental Gerontology* (March 2003), 313–17.

Passarino, G., P. A. Underhill, L. L. Cavalli-Sforza, O. Semino, G. M. Pes, C. Carru, L. Ferrucci, et al. "Y Chromosome Binary Markers to Study the High Prevalence of Males in Sardinian Centenarians and the Genetic Structure of the Sardinian Population." *Human Heredity* (September 2001), 136–39.

Pes, G. M., D. Lio, C. Carru, L. Deiana, G. Baggio, C. Franceschi, L. Ferrucci, et al. "Association Between Longevity and Cytokine Gene Polymorphisms: A Study in Sardinian Centenarians." *Aging Clinical And Experimental Research* (June 2004), 244–48.

Pes, G. M., F. Tolu, M. Poulain, A. Errigo, S. Masala, A. Pietrobelli, N. C. Battistini, and M. Maioli. "Lifestyle and Nutrition Related to Male Longevity in Sardinia: An Ecological Study." *Nutrition, Metabolism and Cardiovascular Diseases* (March 2013), 212–19.

Polidori, M. C., E. Mariani, G. Baggio, L. Deiana, C. Carru, G. M. Pes, R. Cecchetti, C. Franceschi, U. Senin, and P. Mecocci. "Different Antioxidant Profiles in Italian Centenarians: The Sardinian Peculiarity." *European Journal of Clinical Nutrition* (July 2007), 922–24.

Poulain, M., G. M. Pes, C. Grasland, C. Carru, L. Ferrucci, G. Baggio, C. Franceschi, and L. Deiana. "Identification of a Geographic Area Characterized by Extreme Longevity in the Sardinia Island: The AKEA study." *Experimental Gerontology* (September 2004), 1423–29.

Poulain, M., G. Pes, and L. Salaris. "A Population Where Men Live as Long as Women: Villagrande Strisaili, Sardinia." *Journal of Aging Research* (2011), article ID 153756, 10 pp.

Tessier, S., and M. Gerber. "Factors Determining the Nutrition Transition in Two Mediterranean Islands: Sardinia and Malta." *Public Health Nutrition* (December 2005), 1286–92.

Universities of Sassari and Cagliari. "New Study Confirms Health Benefits of Pecorino Romano Cheese" [press release]. December 2, 2009. Retrieved from http://www.prnewswire.com/news-releases/new-study-confirms-health-benefits-of-pecorino-romano-cheese-78322487.html.

ADVENTIST

Beezhold, B. L., C. S. Johnston, and D. R. Daigle. "Vegetarian Diets Are Associated With Healthy Mood States: A Cross-Sectional Study in Seventh-Day Adventist Adults." *Nutrition Journal* (2010) 9:26.

Flores-Mateo, G., D. Rojas-Rueda, J. Basora, E. Ros, and J. Salas-Salvadó. "Nut Intake and Adiposity: Meta-Analysis of Clinical Trials." *American Journal of Clinical Nutrition* (June 2013), 1346–55.

Ford, P. A., K. Jaceldo-Siegl, J. W. Lee, W. Youngberg, and S. Tonstad. "Intake of Mediterranean Foods Associated With Positive Affect and Low Negative Affect." *Journal of Psychosomatic Research* (February 2013), 142–48.

Fraser, G. E. "Associations Between Diet and Cancer, Ischemic Heart Disease, and All-Cause Mortality in Non-Hispanic White California Seventh-Day Adventists." *American Journal of Clinical Nutrition* (September 1999), 532S–538S.

Fraser, G. E. "Vegetarian Diets: What Do We Know of Their Effects on Common Chronic Diseases?" *American Journal of Clinical Nutrition* (May 2009), 1607S–1612S.

Fraser, G. E., and D. J. Shavlik. "Risk Factors for All-Cause and Coronary Heart Disease Mortality in the Oldest-Old: The Adventist Health Study." *Archives of Internal Medicine* (October 27, 1997), 2249–58.

Fraser, G. E., and D. J. Shavlik. "Ten Years of Life: Is It a Matter of Choice?" *Archives of Internal Medicine* (July 9, 2001), 1645–52.

Hailu, A., S. F. Knutsen, and G. E. Fraser. "Associations Between Meat Consumption and the Prevalence of Degenerative Arthritis and Soft Tissue Disorders in the Adventist Health Study, California U.S.A." *Journal of Nutrition, Health and Aging* (January–February 2006), 7–14.

Huang, T., B. Yang, J. Zheng, G. Li, M. L. Wahlqvist, and D. Li. "Cardiovascular Disease Mortality and Cancer Incidence in Vegetarians: A Meta-Analysis and Systematic Review." *Annals of Nutrition and Metabolism* (June 2012), 233–40.

Hunt, I. F., N. J. Murphy, and C. Henderson. "Food and Nutrient Intake of Seventh-Day Adventist Women." *American Journal of Clinical Nutrition* (September 1988), 850–51.

Jaceldo-Siegl, K., J. Fan, J. Sabaté, S. F. Knutsen, E. Haddad, W. L. Beeson, R. P. Herring, T. L. Butler, H. Bennett, and G. E. Fraser. "Race-Specific Validation of Food Intake Obtained From a Comprehensive FFQ: The Adventist Health Study-2." *Public Health Nutrition* (November 2011), 1988–97.

Jaceldo-Siegl, K., E. Haddad, K. Oda, G. E. Fraser, and J. Sabaté. "Tree Nuts Are Inversely Associated With Metabolic Syndrome and Obesity: The Adventist Health Study-2." *PLOS ONE* (January 8, 2014), e85133.

Kelly, J. H., Jr., and J. Sabaté. "Nuts and Coronary Heart Disease: An Epidemiological Perspective." *British Journal of Nutrition* (November 2006), S61–67.

Key, T. J., G. E. Fraser, M. Thorogood, P. N. Appleby, V. Beral, G. Reeves, M. L. Burr, et al. "Mortality in Vegetarians and Nonvegetarians: Detailed Findings From a Collaborative Analysis of 5 Prospective Studies." *American Journal of Clinical Nutrition* (September 1999), 516S–524S.

Lousuebsakul-Matthews, V., D. L. Thorpe, R. Knutsen, W. L. Beeson, G. E. Fraser, and S. F. Knutsen. "Legumes and Meat Analogues Consumption Are Associated With Hip Fracture Risk Independently of Meat Intake Among Caucasian Men and Women: The Adventist Health Study-2." *Public Health Nutrition* (Epub October 8, 2013) [ahead of print], 10 pp.

McEvoy, C. T., N. Temple, and J. V. Woodside. "Vegetarian Diets, Low-Meat Diets and Health: A Review." *Public Health Nutrition* (December 2012), 2287–94.

Micha, R., G. Michas, and D. Mozaffarian. "Unprocessed Red and Processed Meats and Risk of Coronary Artery Disease and Type 2 Diabetes: An Updated Review of the Evidence." *Current Atherosclerosis Reports* (December 2012), 515–24.

O'Neil, C. E., D. R. Keast, T. A. Nicklas, and V. L. Fulgoni 3rd. "Nut Consumption Is Associated With Decreased Health Risk Factors for Cardiovascular Disease and Metabolic Syndrome in U.S. Adults: NHANES 1999–2004." *Journal of the American College of Nutrition* (December 2011), 502–10.

Orlich, M. J., P. N. Singh, J. Sabaté, K. Jaceldo-Siegl, J. Fan, S. Knutsen, W. L. Beeson, and G. E. Fraser. "Vegetarian Dietary Patterns and Mortality in Adventist Health Study 2." *JAMA Internal Medicine* (July 8, 2013), 1230–38.

Pettersen, B. J., R. Anousheh, J. Fan, K. Jaceldo-Siegl, and G. E. Fraser. "Vegetarian Diets and Blood Pressure Among White Subjects: Results From the Adventist Health Study-2 (AHS-2)." *Public Health Nutrition* (October 2012), 1909–16.

Rizzo, N. S., K. Jaceldo-Siegl, J. Sabaté, and G. E. Fraser. "Nutrient Profiles of Vegetarian and Nonvegetarian Dietary Patterns." *Journal of the Academy of Nutrition and Dietetics* (December 2013), 1610–19.

Rizzo, N. S., J. Sabaté, K. Jaceldo-Siegl, and G. E. Fraser. "Vegetarian Dietary Patterns Are Associated With a Lower Risk of Metabolic Syndrome: The Adventist Health Study 2." *Diabetes Care* (May 2011), 1225–27.

Ros, E., L. C. Tapsell, and J. Sabaté. "Nuts and Berries for Heart Health." *Current Atherosclerosis Reports* (November 2010), 397–406.

Sabaté, J. "Nut Consumption, Vegetarian Diets, Ischemic Heart Disease Risk, and All-Cause Mortality: Evidence From Epidemiologic Studies." *American Journal of Clinical Nutrition* (September 1999), 500S–503S.

Sabaté, J., K. Oda, and E. Ros. "Nut Consumption and Blood Lipid Levels: A Pooled Analysis of 25 Intervention Trials." *Archives of Internal Medicine* (May 10, 2010), 821–27.

Singh, P. N., E. Haddad, S. Tonstad, and G. E. Fraser. "Does Excess Body Fat Maintained After the Seventh Decade Decrease Life Expectancy?" *Journal of the American Geriatric Society* (June 2011), 1003–11.

Singh, P. N., J. Sabaté, and G. E. Fraser. "Does Low Meat Consumption Increase Life Expectancy in Humans?" *American Journal of Clinical Nutrition* (September 2003), 526S–532S.

Tantamango-Bartley, Y., K. Jaceldo-Siegl, J. Fan, and G. Fraser. "Vegetarian Diets and the Incidence of Cancer in a Low-Risk Population." *Cancer Epidemiology Biomarkers and Prevention* (February 2013), 286–94.

Tantamango, Y. M., S. F. Knutsen, L. Beeson, G. Fraser, and J. Sabaté. "Association Between Dietary Fiber and Incident Cases of Colon Polyps: The Adventist Health Study." *Gastrointestinal Cancer Research* (September 2011), 161–67.

Tantamango, Y. M., S. F. Knutsen, W. L. Beeson, G. Fraser, and J. Sabaté. "Foods and Food Groups Associated With the Incidence of Colorectal Polyps: The Adventist Health Study." *Nutrition and Cancer* (May 2011), 565–72.

Tonstad, S., T. Butler, R. Yan, and G. E. Fraser. "Type of Vegetarian Diet, Body Weight, and Prevalence of Type 2 Diabetes." *Diabetes Care* (May 2009), 791–96.

Tonstad, S., N. Malik, and E. Haddad. "A High-Fibre Bean-Rich Diet Versus a Low-Carbohydrate Diet for Obesity." *Journal of Human Nutrition and Dietetics* (Epub April 30, 2013) [ahead of print].

Tonstad, S., K. Stewart, K. Oda, M. Batech, R. P. Herring, and G. E. Fraser. "Vegetarian Diets and Incidence of Diabetes in the Adventist Health Study-2." *Nutrition, Metabolism and Cardiovascular Diseases* (April 2013), 292–99.

Vang, A., P. N. Singh, J. W. Lee, E. H. Haddad, and C. H. Brinegar. "Meats, Processed Meats, Obesity, Weight Gain and Occurrence of Diabetes Among Adults: Findings From Adventist Health Studies." *Annals of Nutrition and Metabolism* (May 2008), 96–104.

Wang, Y., M. A. Beydoun, B. Caballero, T. L. Gary, and R. Lawrence. "Trends and Correlates in Meat Consumption Patterns in the U.S. Adult Population." *Public Health Nutrition* (September 2010), 1333–45.

COSTA RICA

Bazzano, L. A., J. He, L. G. Ogden, C. Loria, S. Vupputuri, L. Myers, and P. K. Whelton. "Legume Consumption and Risk of Coronary Heart Disease in U.S. Men and Women: NHANES I Epidemiologic Follow-Up Study." *Archives of Internal Medicine* (November 26, 2001), 2573–78.

Bazzano, L. A., A. M. Thompson, M. T. Tees, C. H. Nguyen, and D. M. Winham. "Non-Soy Legume Consumption Lowers Cholesterol Levels: A Meta-Analysis of Randomized Controlled Trials." *Nutrition, Metabolism and Cardiovascular Diseases* (February 2011), 94–103.

Darmadi-Blackberry, I., M. L. Wahlqvist, A. Kouris-Blazos, B. Steen, W. Lukito, Y. Horie, and K. Horie. "Legumes: The Most Important Dietary Predictor of Survival in Older People of Different Ethnicities." *Asia Pacific Journal of Clinical Nutrition* (June 2004), 217–20.

Davinelli, S., D. C. Willcox, and G. Scapagnini. "Extending Healthy Ageing: Nutrient-Sensitive Pathway and Centenarian Population." *Immunity and Ageing* (2012) 9:9.

Flores, M. "Food Patterns in Central America and Panama." In *Tradition, Science and Practice in Dietetics: Proceedings of the International Congress of Dietetics, July 10–14, 1961.* Newman Books, 1961.

Flores, M., and J. Aranas-Pastor. "Evaluacion dietetica a nivel nacional en Costa Rica: combios de una decada." *Archivos Latinoamericanos de Nutrición* (September 1980), 432–50.

Hutchins, A. M., D. M. Winham, and S. V. Thompson. "Phaseolus Beans: Impact on Glycaemic Response and Chronic Disease Risk in Human Subjects." *British Journal of Nutrition* (August 2012), S52–65.

Institute of Nutrition of Central America and Panama (INCAP) and the Interdepartmental Committee on Nutrition for National Development (ICNND). Tables 3, 4, and 106. In *Nutritional Evaluation of the Population of Central America and Panama, 1965–1967.*

Mollard, R. C., A. Zykus, B. L. Luhovyy, M. F. Nunez, C. L. Wong, and G. H. Anderson. "The Acute Effects of a Pulse-Containing Meal on Glycaemic Responses and Measures of Satiety and Satiation Within and At a Later Meal." *British Journal of Nutrition* (August 2012), 509–17.

Rebello, C. J., F. L. Greenway, and J. W. Finley. "A Review of the Nutritional Value of Legumes and Their Effects on Obesity and Its Related Co-Morbidities." *Obesity Review* (Epub January 17, 2014) [ahead of print].

Rehkopf, D. H., W. H. Dow, L. Rosero-Bixby, J. Lin, E. S. Epel, and E. H. Blackburn. "Longer Leukocyte Telomere Length in Costa Rica's Nicoya Peninsula: A Population-Based Study." *Experimental Gerontology* (November 2013), 1266–73.

Rosero-Bixby, L. "The Exceptionally High Life Expectancy of Costa Rican Nonagenarians." *Demography* (August 2008), 673–91.

Rosero-Bixby, L., and W. H. Dow. "Predicting Mortality With Biomarkers: A Population-Based Prospective Cohort Study for Elderly Costa Ricans." *Population Health Metrics* (2012) 10:11.

Rosero-Bixby, L., W. H. Dow, and A. Laclé. "Insurance and Other Socioeconomic Determinants of Elderly Longevity in a Costa Rican Panel." *Journal of Biosocial Science* (November 2005), 705–20.

Thompson, S. V., D. M. Winham, and A. M. Hutchins. "Bean and Rice Meals Reduce Postprandial Glycemic Response in Adults With Type 2 Diabetes: A Cross-Over Study." *Nutrition Journal* (2012) 11:23.

Index

Index

OTHER BOOKS BY **DAN BUETTNER**

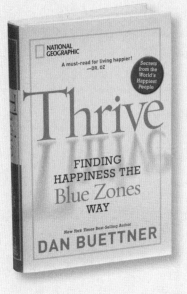

Dan Buettner reports on the surprising findings from his five-year global study on the keys to personal happiness. He examines the unique lifestyles of the happiest people on the planet and explains how to integrate these vital habits into our own lives.

"Dan Buettner has found the world's happiest places and brought back the secrets to living a fulfilling life. The guide tells us exactly what changes we need to make— and best of all, they're easy."—Dr. Oz

"In addition to sharing his extraordinary accounts of the happiest people on the planet, Buettner details how to incorporate these powerful characteristics into our daily routine so that we, too, can thrive."—*Psychology Today*

In this *New York Times* bestseller (featured on *Oprah*) Dan Buettner travels the globe to uncover the top strategies for longevity found in the Blue Zones— places in the world where higher percentages of people enjoy remarkably long, full lives. He discloses the recipe, blending this unique lifestyle formula with the latest scientific findings to inspire easy, lasting change that may add years to your life.

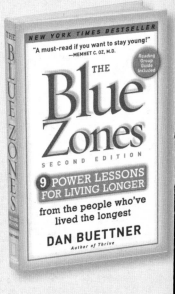

"[Buettner] would like to draw a big blue circle around the entire USA."—*USA Today*

"Dan Buettner has gathered some of the top scientists in the world to study so-called blue zones. He wrote the book about these remarkable places where it's been proven people tend to live longer."—*NBC News*

AVAILABLE WHEREVER BOOKS ARE SOLD and at nationalgeographic.com/book

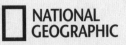 **NATIONAL GEOGRAPHIC**

 Like us on Facebook: Nat Geo Books
Follow us on Twitter: @NatGeoBooks